Contents

Other Health Books by Roger Mason

Lower Blood Pressure Without Drugs

Lower Your Cholesterol Without Drugs

The Minerals You Need

The Natural Diabetes Cure

The Natural Prostate Cure

The Supplements You Need

Testosterone Is Your Friend

What Is Beta Glucan?

Zen Macrobiotics for Americans

Introduction

Women in Western countries, particularly the United States, are at risk for an inordinate amount of health problems. Heart disease, diabetes, osteoporosis, arthritis, Alzheimer's, obesity, and many other diseases are affecting women in unprecedented numbers. Cancer rates are also on the rise; one in eight women will be diagnosed with breast cancer, and one in three women will undergo a hysterectomy. Stages of the female cycle are now thought of as medical conditions instead of natural processes, as symptoms of premenstrual syndrome and menopause have become more severe and often debilitating. What is the reason behind the decline in women's health? More importantly, how can we reverse this trend?

While many factors contribute to disease, the two most basic are diet and lifestyle. A diet high in fat and sugar—which is all too common among the Western population, and Americans in particular—in combination with a sedentary lifestyle, alcohol consumption, smoking, and various other factors lead to medical conditions. More specifically, they lead to hormone imbalance, which is the root of practically every chronic disease. Your hormones must work together to carry out vital functions. Therefore, when even one is thrown out of balance, several processes can be negatively affected. Unfortunately, the mainstream medical community's answer to this problem has been unnatural hormones, such as horse estrogen and synthetic progestins, as well as unnecessary invasive procedures like hysterectomy. These methods—which are often prescribed without even first testing hormone levels—usually only cause further harm and create new problems. Women are rarely informed about bioidentical hormones, which have proven benefits, and instead given pharmaceutical drugs that merely target the symptoms rather than address the underlying cause. These also have a number of adverse side effects and health risks that may prove to be just as bad—if not worse—than the condition being treated. The combination of an unhealthy diet and lifestyle, hormone imbalance, and inadequate "treatments" is the basis of disease and the reason behind the health crisis facing women today. All of these health issues culminate in menopause, which, for most women, is now spent dealing with undesirable symptoms and medical conditions rather than enjoying a new phase of their lives.

But it does not have to be this way. There are steps you can take to prevent and eliminate the causes of disease instead of merely covering up the symptoms with ineffective treatments. You can treat and even reverse medical conditions naturally through diet and lifestyle instead of taking prescription drugs or undergoing risky medical procedures. You can be in control of your health and welfare. You can change your destiny.

Natural Health for Women, an updated version of my book *No More Horse Estrogen!,* is a comprehensive guide to holistic health based on several decades of clinical research. In addition to information that cannot be found anywhere else, this unique book gives you the tools and knowledge you need to naturally prevent, treat, and reverse a wide range of medical conditions, from arthritis to diabetes. The book opens with a chapter on menopause, the time in a woman's life when many health issues often culminate all at once. These issues usually have their origin in hormone imbalance and the toxic therapies designed to treat it—topics explored in the next several chapters. *Natural Health for Women* also takes a close look at each of the major diseases on the rise today in the United States and other Western countries, and clearly explains how they can be treated with a natural whole-foods diet, proven nutritional supplements, natural hormone balance, regular exercise, and fasting, among other health-promoting practices. Finally, the book tells you about the vitamins, minerals, and other nutrients that are essential to your health, and how much you should take in order to reinforce the positive effects of a healthy diet and lifestyle.

Good health is real wealth, and by choosing a holistic lifestyle, you can enjoy a long, happy, and healthy life. There is no naturopathic or life-extension doctor who alone can do this for you. *You* must help yourself by being responsible and proactive when it comes to matters of your health, and reading *Natural Health for Women* is an important first step.

1. Menopause

In 1839, a Frenchman by the name of C.F. Menville became the first person to write a book entirely about menopause. In it he wrote, "When the vital forces seek to work together in the interest of the uterus, they go to join those of the mind and the rest of the body. The critical age passed, women have the hope of a longer life than men, [and] their thought acquires more precision, more scope and vitality." This pleasantly enlightened view of the natural changes through which every woman goes contrasts very strongly with the prevalent view in Western society today—namely, that menopause is an uncomfortable and often distressing process accompanied by adverse symptoms and side effects, and one that marks the loss of womanhood, not a new phase of it.

Today in the United States, there are nearly 40 million menopausal women, and another 30 million women of the baby boomer generation are approaching menopause. Since women are now living longer—the average life expectancy is 78 in the United States—more than one-third of their lives will be lived after menopause. Think about that. Women are postmenopausal for more than half of their adult lives. There is no reason why this time should not be enjoyed—and it can, provided that you follow a healthy lifestyle in the years leading up to, during, and following menopause.

This book is designed to help you do this, but first you should have a firm understanding of menopause and its place in the female life cycle. This chapter provides an overview of menopause, highlighting the symptoms, associated medical conditions, and dominant attitude towards this natural life stage in Western culture. By exploring the question of why menopause is perceived as a negative experience, you will see how changing your attitude and general lifestyle is the solution.

WHAT IS MENOPAUSE?

Menopause is generally defined as the time in a woman's life when the body goes through hormonal changes that result in the cessation of the menstrual cycle, meaning that she can no longer become pregnant. Typically, this process begins between the ages of forty-five and fifty-five, though it can begin as early as the late thirties or early forties. (In the United States, most women have their last period at the age of fifty-two.) Menopause is considered to be complete when a woman goes twelve months without getting her period. The time leading up to this point is called *perimenopause,* also referred to as premenopause or the climacteric, which can last for months or several years. During this time, women may experience a number of physical changes caused by hormonal imbalances, such as estrogen dominance—an imbalanced ratio between the primary female hormones, estrogen and progesterone. The impact that these hormones have on your body, especially when levels become unbalanced, is discussed in more detail in the next few chapters (see pages 9, 17, and 23). Certain lifestyle factors—including poor diet, obesity, lack of exercise, and taking prescription drugs—may also intensify the symptoms of perimenopause.

The spectrum of experience is wide when it comes to perimenopause. While some women may breeze through this time and experience minimal, if any, symptoms, others have endless difficulties. However, a hallmark of perimenopause that most women experience is menstrual irregularity, which is characterized by periods that are longer or shorter in duration, occasional skipped periods or spotting, and heavier or lighter menstrual flow. Periods usually become less and less frequent until they stop altogether. Additional symptoms of perimenopause include:

- Changes in mood, including increased anxiety, irritability, and depression

- Dental problems

- Digestive disturbances

- Fatigue

- Forgetfulness

- Headaches

- Hot flashes

- Increased vaginal infections and/or vaginal dryness

- Joint pain

- Night sweats

- Reduced sex drive and/or sexual satisfaction

- Sleep problems or insomnia, which may be caused by hot flashes

- Urinary incontinence

There are also several medical conditions associated with menopause—all of which will be discussed later in this book—including cardiovascular problems, increased cholesterol levels, and bone loss. Bone loss, which usually begins before menopause and worsens over time, stems from decreasing levels of progesterone and androgens, and raises the risk of osteoporosis (see page 69). These health problems in combination with the symptoms listed above help to explain why menopause is generally viewed as an illness or disease. Interestingly, though, this attitude is held primarily by Western industrialized nations, where menopause is usually accompanied by unpleasant side effects and numerous other problems.

MENOPAUSE IN WESTERN CULTURE

In contrast to women in Western society, including the United States, females in less developed countries experience far fewer problems as they approach menopause, which is due mainly to their healthier diet and lifestyle. To deal with the unpleasant problems associated with menopause, the standard medical treatment up until 2003 was hormone replacement therapy (HRT), which was intended to replace the female hormones in which menopausal women were supposedly deficient, in turn alleviating side effects. However, this procedure often involved the use of substances like horse estrogen, artificial progestins, and mind-numbing drugs like Valium and Prozac, which were found to have undesirable side effects and a number of health consequences, including some types of cancer. Clinical trials of certain agents used in HRT also found an increased risk of heart disease, blood clots, and stroke.

Despite the risks, HRT is still used. Some doctors give women powerful substances like horse estrogen without even testing their natural levels of hormones like estradiol, estrone, estriol, DHEA, testosterone, pregnenolone, melatonin, growth hormone (GH), or thyroid hormones (T3 and T4). The fact that HRT continues to be used in conventional medicine ignores current science and causes even more problems than it purports to cure. The serious side effects and increased number of medical issues caused by HRT are rarely, if ever, discussed. Yet, under this treatment, women just get worse and worse, and many choose to stop the therapy. In fact, estrogen supplements are rarely necessary, since the vast majority of Western women (both pre- and postmenopausal) have very high levels of the estrogens estradiol and estrone (see pages 12 and 13).

Considering all the problems Western women experience during menopause—whether due to lifestyle factors or harmful treatments like HRT—it's no wonder that the predominant Western view of it is very negative. A stage that should be thought of as a very normal, desirable, and natural part of a woman's life is instead looked upon with fear and dread. This fear stems in part from the belief that menopause marks the end of physical attractiveness and sexual satisfaction, as well as physical and mental health. In addition, menopause is regarded as being synonymous with aging, which also tends to be viewed negatively in Western culture.

Because women face more social pressure than men to look a certain way, they may feel more of a sense of loss when they begin to age. However, it's important to keep in mind that this is not so much a loss as it is a change. Life does not always remain as it was in your twenties—and this is not a bad thing. Across all cultures, men and women alike may experience a decrease in sexual enjoyment and performance as they age. But instead of mourning this decline, aging should be seen as an opportunity to find other sources of enjoyment and fulfillment. Sex is not the "be-all and end-all" of existence, and entering a more mature life stage is a chance to discover and appreciate other aspects of life.

The second part of women's apprehension about menopause—the perceived decline of their mental and physical abilities—also needs to be addressed. Due to the unhealthy lifestyle followed by a significant portion of the Western population, serious medical issues are on the rise among adults, both male and female. Of course, declining mental and physical health is a natural part of the aging process in all cultures, but the deterioration is much more dramatic in Western society. But as the saying goes, an ounce of prevention is worth ten pounds of cure. Instead of viewing medical problems—especially those associated with menopause—as inevitable, nip them in the bud by adopting a healthy lifestyle while you are young. This means choosing better foods, starting a full supplement program, balancing your hormones, eliminating bad habits like smoking, and exercising regularly. It is advised that you fast one day per week and, whenever possible, stop prescription medications for conditions that can be treated naturally. Adopting these lifestyle practices earlier in life will allow menopause to become a time for practicing holistic living rather than trying to eliminate one health issue after the next.

Finally, since menopause typically occurs in middle or late-middle age, many women consider it synonymous with being "over the hill." In Western culture, older people are generally viewed as being less valuable and useful. Yet, this is not the case in other societies around the world, where mature adults—particularly women—are appreciated and respected. They are seen as sources of wisdom, good judgment, humor, advice, insight, compassion, and experience. The matriarchs are society's honored storytellers, healers, advisers, and sages. Maturity is regarded as an asset with many advantages, not a liability.

If this attitude was embraced in our culture as well, much of the anxiety caused by menopause would be greatly reduced, if not eliminated outright. After all, getting older is simply a matter of taking on a new role in society—it does not make anyone less important. In Western culture, however, there is an unconscious obsession with the idea of living forever, as well as a reluctance to accept the idea of mortality. This engrained fear makes it difficult to enjoy the aging process, which should be a positive time of spiritual growth, development, and transformation. There is no better time for self-development and relaxation than your later years. This is the time to truly enjoy your life instead of worrying about your career, paying your bills, or making money. It is a perfect time to do charity or philanthropic work, volunteer, and contribute to your community. This is the chance to realize that we are, in essence, spiritual beings beyond both birth and death. Nothing is more important than personal development and spiritual realization, and entering this new life stage is an opportunity to focus on these pursuits.

In sum, it is possible to avoid the major health problems that are responsible for the negative view of menopause in Western society. The medical conditions and illnesses that frequently accompany menopause and postmenopause in Western industrialized countries are not normal—no matter how predominant they may be—and they should not be seen as inevitable. Less than 100 years ago, premenstrual syndrome (PMS), sexual dysfunction, osteoporosis, various cancers, Alzheimer's, dementia, arthritis, diabetes, stroke, heart disease, senility, and unwanted menopausal symptoms were not the common ailments that they are today. This just goes to show that such conditions are certainly not inherent, normal, or unavoidable. They simply do not have to happen, and with the right lifestyle choices, they can be prevented.

CONCLUSION

The Western lifestyle has become increasingly unhealthy over the past century. As a result, menopause, as well as aging in general, is now a burden on women's health instead of a process that is celebrated and appreciated. But now, with our ever-expanding knowledge of health, hygiene, nutrition, biology, and other sciences, we can and should be enjoying healthier lives than we were 100 years ago. We may be living longer, but the quality of these extra years is worse. Longevity without a parallel quality of life is pointless.

It is said that "youth is wasted on the young," and there is a lot of truth to this statement. After menopause, wisdom, serenity, and appreciation for life is enhanced. The last third of your life can be the most enjoyable period of all; it can be a time of creativity, self-development, and good health, rather than declining health and independence. It can and should be a time of personal fulfillment, discovering new hobbies, introspection, and leisure. To make this possible, you must first adopt a healthy lifestyle—and the sooner the better. The following chapters will give you the information and guidance you need to make smart lifestyle choices that promote optimal wellness. This will ensure that menopause, as well as aging in general, will be spent enjoying life in a natural, healthy way. As you will see, it all comes down to natural hormone balance.

2. Estrogen and Hormone Replacement Therapy

As you read in the last chapter, there are many misconceptions about menopause in Western society. Perhaps the most significant is that menopause causes a drop in a woman's level of estrogen, the primary and most frequently discussed female *hormone*—a chemical substance that delivers important information to cells so that vital functions can be performed. This fallacy is the driving force behind hormone replacement therapy (HRT), a dangerous and toxic treatment that is correlated with many serious medical conditions, including cancer and cardiovascular disease. This chapter explores the history of hormone replacement therapy, which was originally touted as a "cure" for menopause. It also outlines the three primary forms of human estrogen, as well as types that are not naturally made by the body. This will help you to better understand why natural hormone balance is so critically important to your overall health.

THE HISTORY OF HORMONE REPLACEMENT THERAPY (HRT)

Although estrogen replacement therapy (ERT) was approved by the US Food and Drug Administration (FDA) as a treatment for menopause in 1941, it did not become a highly publicized and hugely profitable industry until the 1960s. This success was due to its promotion by pharmaceutical corporations, as well as doctors like Robert Wilson, who saw the therapy as a "cure" for menopause. Wilson, a gynecologist, wrote a book entitled *Feminine Forever* in 1966, in which he stated that menopause was a disease characterized by estrogen insufficiency that required treatment. He claimed that while the condition marked the end of women's femininity, it could be prevented by taking estrogen, specifically horse estrogen extracted from pregnant mares. The book *Now! The Pills to Keep Women Young!* by Ann Walsh, which was published around the same time, also advocated horse estrogen as a solution for menopause.

Despite the fact that these books were completely undocumented and scientifically unsound, they were monumental successes. Pharmaceutical corporations that profited from the popularity of hormone replacement drugs were even more successful. But their success was also baseless, since there was no evidence that menopausal women were even estrogen deficient in the first place, let alone that estrogen supplementation had actual benefits. The use of horse estrogen instead of human bioidentical estrogens was prima facie insanity, but that didn't stop women from taking it or doctors from prescribing it.

Estrogen replacement therapy hit a roadblock in 1975 when the *New England Journal of Medicine* published a study showing increased cancer rates among women who had used estrogen drugs—including increased uterine cancer rates of up to 800 percent—among many other problems. But instead of removing estrogen from the market, manufacturers instead added progestin analogs—synthetic progesterone—to estrogen drugs in a supposed effort to reduce health risks. In reality, however, this was done purely for profit, since natural hormones cannot be patented. Furthermore, although progestins are completely unnatural, many doctors used the words "progestin" and "progesterone" interchangeably as they continue to do today, misleading patients as a result.

Therefore, *estrogen* replacement therapy became *hormone* replacement therapy (HRT), but the side effects were every bit as severe as before. Hormone replacement therapy did not fulfill the many promises made, and its side effects were simply intolerable. In other words, HRT was a dismal failure. Most women did not refill their estrogen prescriptions, and only very rarely did they report any benefits. Nevertheless, doctors continued to relentlessly prescribe it to their female patients. Finally, in 2002, the findings of the Women's Health Initiative study revealed once and for all that hormone replacement therapy was harmful, raising the risk of not only uterine cancer but also breast cancer, stroke, heart attack, blood clots, and many other serious medical problems. Yet, this has not brought an end to HRT, as the medical field has stopped short of deeming it too toxic to use.

HRT AND MENOPAUSE

The larger medical fallacy underlying the problem of hormone replacement therapy is the idea that women's estrogen levels drop as a result of menopause, and that these low levels are directly responsible for the negative symptoms, from hot flashes to depression. Countless clinical studies have shown quite the opposite. As stated in Chapter 1, women in Western countries tend to be very high in estrogen, particularly the estrogens estradiol and estrone (see pages 12 and 13), even after menopause. While it is true that levels of estriol (see page 14), progesterone, pregnenolone, melatonin, thyroid hormones T3 and T4, DHEA, and testosterone can decrease during and after menopause, doctors almost never measure these levels. Nor do they test women's levels of estradiol and estrone. If they did, they would know that estrogen supplementation is rarely necessary for most American and European women.

In general, Western women have high estradiol and estrone levels due to eating a diet high in calories and fat, and low in fiber. Low levels of omega-3s, lack of exercise, alcohol intake, and excess weight are also influential factors. By contrast, women in agrarian (non-industrialized) countries, as well as many Asian countries, have lower estrogen levels. They also do not experience high rates of cancer, heart disease, osteoporosis, arthritis, undesirable symptoms like hot flashes, and other problems that afflict so many Western women.

Therefore, it is clear that menopause is anything but a disease caused by low estrogen levels and cured by supplementing with estrogen, particularly estradiol and estrone. Moreover, using estrogen extracted from horses is simply irrational, especially since modern science has given us forms of estrogen that are *bioidentical*—biochemically the same as—human estrogen. The many medical studies that have been done on postmenopausal women show that their levels of estrone and estradiol do fall somewhat, but just enough to prevent menstruation and fertilization. After menopause, estrogen levels are sufficient to perform all the other necessary functions. In other words, the female body is biologically programmed so that fertility ends without affecting the body's other vital processes.

Menopause is an important and necessary part of the natural order of life. Doctors would do immeasurable good for women by testing the levels of *all* their basic hormones and keeping them in balance as much as possible. Fortunately, you don't have to go to an endocrinologist, gynecologist, or even your family doctor to do so. Now you can accurately and scientifically test most of your own hormone levels with inexpensive saliva test kits without a prescription. Other levels can be measured by blood testing services offered through Internet-based companies. Since having control over your hormone metabolism and overall health is vitally important, measuring your hormone levels without a doctor is a topic that is covered in more detail in Chapter 5 (see page 29). However, women who have had hysterectomies should practice extra caution, as discussed in Chapter 7 (see page 48).

Hormones affect both your body and mind, and keeping them in balance is central to your longevity and general well-being. The next section takes a look at the hormone at the center of the controversy that has been discussed so far: estrogen.

WHAT IS ESTROGEN?

The term *estrogen* actually refers to not one hormone, but a group of similar hormones that are produced mainly in the ovaries, and in the adrenal glands and fat tissues in smaller amounts. Men also produce estrogen, but its role in the male body is not clear. In females, estrogen regulates development and reproduction, as well as various metabolic processes like cholesterol management and bone growth. There are seven natural estrogens in the human body, but the three primary ones are *estrone* (E1), *estradiol* (E2), and *estriol* (E3). These substances are present in different amounts in the body and have slightly different roles.

Estrone (E1)

Estrone, which normally comprises only about 5 to 10 percent of human estrogen, is the second-most powerful estrogen. In terms of hormone therapy, estrone is a stronger form of estrogen than estriol, but weaker than estradiol. The prevailing medical belief is that women are deficient in estrone, but this is a fallacy; in reality, estrone deficiencies are very uncommon. Women in Western countries, including the United States, actually have excessive estrone due to factors such as obesity (see page 98), which affects approximately one-third of American women, and high-fat diets. According to recent estimates, fats make up 42 percent of the calories in an average American's diet, with saturated ("bad") fat making up between one-third and one-half of those fats. Estrone can be reduced by following a diet high in fiber and low in fat, losing weight, exercising, avoiding alcohol, and taking nutritional supplements like DIM and flaxseed oil (see pages 119 and 120). Anti-aromatase drugs (aromatase inhibitors), which are often prescribed to postmenopausal women to lower estrogen levels, should not be used, as they are dangerous and can cause a number of adverse side effects, including bone loss and cardiovascular problems.

You can test your estrone level with an inexpensive at-home saliva testing kit. You should consider taking estrone only if your level is low, but never take oral forms, which are poorly absorbed and may produce harmful metabolites when taken in large doses. Instead, use bioidentical hormones, which are molecularly identical to natural hormones. Bioidentical estrone can be *transdermal*—a topical gel or cream applied directly to the skin—or *sublingual*, meaning that it is taken under the tongue. The sublingual method is far more effective, however, since it allows for better absorption into the bloodstream. About 99 percent of the hormone is absorbed when taken sublingually, but only 20 percent is absorbed when it is used transdermally. If your estrone is low, take 0.1 mg (100 mcg) sublingually every day, or apply 0.5 mg of cream or gel to your skin. Just keep the difference in absorption in mind.

Estradiol (E2)

Although estradiol, like estrone, accounts for only 5 to 10 percent of human estrogen, it is the strongest type. When used in hormone therapy, estradiol is twelve times more potent than estrone, and a full eighty times more potent than estriol. Menopausal women are often told by their physicians that they are low in estradiol and need to take supplements despite not having had their hormone levels tested. But as with estrone, both pre-menopausal and postmenopausal women—particularly in the United States—are very high in estradiol, which is due to factors like obesity and excessive consumption of saturated fats. Therefore, most women should be trying to reduce their levels, not raise them.

Estradiol is one of the main components of horse estrogen—also called conjugated equine estrogen—which, until 2002, was the most popular hormone replacement therapy in the world, with an estimated 45 million prescriptions per year. About 50 percent of horse estrogen pharmaceutical products are made up of estradiol and estrone, while the other half consists of equilin and other horse estrogens. Giving women a foreign animal estrogen like equilin is irrational and very dangerous, but as already mentioned, it was a very common practice for decades—and it was done without even first testing a woman's blood levels. In 2002, thanks to the Women's Health Initiative, horse estrogen was finally scientifically discredited and deemed dangerous. Yet, despite the health risks associated with the drug, HRT still uses horse estrogen. The prescription insert made mandatory by the FDA now includes a warning about the risk of breast and uterine cancer, gall bladder disease, abnormal blood clotting, and heart disease, as well as seventeen other side effects.

While horse estrogen should never be used, the small percentage of women who have low estradiol levels can take 0.05 mg (50 mcg) sublingually. Almost all of this amount will be absorbed into the blood. The transdermal method may also be used by applying 0.25 mg (250 mcg) of a cream or gel to the skin. About 50 mcg, or 20 percent, will be absorbed into the blood. Keep in mind that taking bioidentical estradiol sublingually is a more effective method, as it allows for enhanced absorption into the bloodstream. At-home saliva testing kits are inexpensive and readily available, so always measure your hormone levels to make sure you actually have a deficiency before supplementing with estradiol.

Estriol (E3)

Although estriol is the most prominent form of estrogen, making up 80 to 90 percent of the body's supply, little research has been done on it. It is the "forgotten estrogen" that is rarely, if ever, discussed by the mainstream medical community. However, the few studies that have been done on estriol are extremely positive, showing how important it is to female metabolism. Although the biologically weakest form of estrogen, estriol is also the safest and most potentially beneficial. Unlike estrone and estradiol, most women—both premenopausal and postmenopausal—are deficient in estriol, and 100 percent of obese women have low levels. At Fujita Health University in Japan (*Nippon Naibunpi Gakkai Zasshi* v. 72, 1996), doctors studied obese women and found that literally all of them were low in estriol—not just most of them, but *all* of them. Unfortunately, estriol is not manufactured in the United States, sold in US pharmacies, or listed in pharmacy source-books. Estriol creams are available on the Internet, but they tend to be overpriced and contain only about 50 mg per unit. The label on a 2-ounce jar or tube of estriol cream should state that it contains approximately 150 mg (0.25 percent) of natural USP estriol, which means that the product has been approved by the US Pharmacopeial Convention. You can find good-quality estriol creams online for only about twenty dollars. Never take oral forms of estriol as they are poorly absorbed by the body and broken down into unwanted metabolites. You should also stay away from homeopathic estriol creams, which are useless and ineffective.

Always make sure that you have low estriol levels before taking supplements. You can self-administer a saliva test to measure your levels or have your blood tested by a doctor. Keep in mind that blood tests administered by a health-care professional can be costly, while at-home testing kits are convenient, inexpensive, and readily available. Also be aware that estriol levels fluctuate all the time—even throughout the day—so it's important that you note the time of day when you take the test. If you find that you are deficient in estriol, take bioidentical hormones only in the form of sublingual drops or a topical (transdermal) cream. When using a topical cream or gel, use one-quarter teaspoon of a 0.25 percent product (150 mg per 2-ounce jar). This puts about 3 mg on your skin and about 0.6

mg (600 mcg), or 2 percent, into your blood. Because the dose is slightly higher, you can use this six days a week instead of seven.

More research should be done on estriol in the future so that doctors become more aware of its importance. Hopefully one day, American companies will produce estriol creams, gels, and sublingual drops, and make this natural hormone readily available for women. Estriol is discussed in more detail in Chapter 3 (see page 17).

Other Estrogens

In addition to the estrogens naturally produced by the body, there are a few other types that should be mentioned as well. First, there is *ethinyl estradiol*, the main estrogen used in most birth control pills. This is a completely synthetic estrogen derived from human estradiol (E2), but it is much more potent and, therefore, very dangerous. There is a long list of precautions, drug interactions, and adverse side effects associated with oral contraceptives containing ethinyl estradiol. There are also many short- and long-term health risks, including blood clots, heart attack, and some types of cancer.

Selective estrogen receptor modulators (SERMs) are another dangerous form of synthetic estrogen. Also called "designer estrogens," SERMs are prescription drugs that can take different actions on different tissues in the body, either turning on or turning off estrogen receptors. Their complex mechanism of action is not well understood, and they have destabilizing toxic effects. Since their activity is similar to estrogen, SERMs can have harmful consequences, such as an increased risk of breast cancer. SERMs should never be used under any circumstances, as they may be even worse for you than horse estrogen and progestins. Aromatase inhibitors, which act similarly to SERMs and are frequently used to lower estrogen levels, should also not be used.

Finally, *phytoestrogens* and *xenoestrogens,* substances that are said to mimic estrogen, should be mentioned. It is a widely held myth that plants contain hormone-like compounds called "phytoestrogens." Health practitioners and scientists alike have claimed that these plant pigments have estrogen-like activity. They do not. No plant has hormone-mimicking activity or hormone-like compounds. Soy isoflavones are very beneficial substances with many health benefits, but they are unrelated to hormones in every way. They have nothing to do with estrogen or any other hormone, either chemically or biologically. Hormones exist only in animals, not in plants. Remember, not every claim made by scientists is a fact. Remember, scientists also once told us that vitamin E was not necessary for nutrition, and that hydrogenated (trans) fats were not harmful.

There is a similar fallacy regarding *xenoestrogens* ("foreign estrogen"), which are supposedly environmental toxins that mimic estrogen and attach to estrogen receptors in the body. It is widely claimed that these chemicals are found in pesticides and fertilizers, plastics, household cleaners, food preservatives and dyes, among other substances with which people come into regular contact. Certainly, there are many environmental pollutants and poisons that we cannot avoid, but none of them at all have anything to do with estrogen or any other hormone. Hormones are secreted by mammals, not by plants and factories.

While natural estrogen is required for the body to function properly, it can be detrimental if it is taken when the body is not deficient. Moreover, synthetic forms of estrogen are downright dangerous, and should never be used. Women should measure their hormones to determine their estrogen levels, and supplement only if they have an insufficiency—which is a rare occurrence in Western countries. It is important to have your estrogen levels tested regularly and monitor the progress of bioidentical hormone therapy.

CONCLUSION

Just because a belief is widely held does not make it a fact, and this is certainly true in the case of hormone replacement therapy, as well as the predominant attitude towards menopause in Western society. Contrary to what most people assume, menopause is not synonymous with low estrogen levels. Moreover, "therapy" with non-human or synthetic estrogen is *not* beneficial—it is the opposite. This is why it is so critical that you take responsibility for your health and learn the facts about hormone balance and hormone therapy. You owe it to yourself to measure your hormone levels regularly, which can now be done from the convenience of your home. You should also find a doctor who understands the importance of natural hormone balance and will prescribe only bioidentical hormones—not harmful horse estrogen or synthetic pharmaceutical products. Natural hormone balance is essential to your health.

3. Estriol—
The Forgotten Estrogen

Although it has been largely ignored by the mainstream medical community, estriol (E3) is the most potentially beneficial estrogen, which is why it deserves its own chapter. One of the three primary human estrogens highlighted in Chapter 2, estriol is the most abundant estrogen in the human body, accounting for about 80 percent of the total estrogen supply. Estriol also has the weakest effects compared to that of estrone and estradiol. While this trait has, perhaps, made it seem insignificant, estriol is actually the most important and beneficial type. In addition to being the safest form of estrogen, estriol has most protective and health-promoting effects. This chapter takes a closer look at this "forgotten" hormone and explains why estriol should be taken more seriously, both as a component of bioidentical hormone replacement therapy and as a vital element in your overall health and well-being.

THE BASICS OF ESTRIOL

Despite being the most prominent estrogen, estriol is usually measured only during pregnancy, when it is elevated and thus easier to measure. Blood levels of estriol and other hormones, such as progesterone, increase dramatically during pregnancy to protect the fetus. Low levels of estriol in pregnant women can signal birth defects and other developmental problems, which is why hormone testing is often done periodically over the course of the pregnancy. Estriol levels are rarely measured in non-pregnant women, who actually tend to be deficient in the hormone—especially women over forty in the United States and other Western countries. Deficiencies have also been seen in teenage girls, particularly those who are overweight. The prevalence of estriol insufficiency among non-pregnant Western women is due to factors like obesity, lack of exercise, and a diet high in saturated fats. Men, however, are hardly ever deficient in estriol.

Low estriol levels are rarely acknowledged or discussed by most health-care professionals, let alone treated as a health concern. Yet, high levels of estriol are beneficial, so taking the necessary steps to raise your level can have many favorable effects. Rural Asian women have higher levels than Western women due to their much healthier diet and lifestyle. Also unlike Western women, rural Asian women have lower levels of estradiol and estrone. Not surprisingly, cancer rates are significantly lower, especially for breast, cervical, ovarian, and uterine cancer. They also suffer far less frequently from diseases like coronary heart disease, osteoporosis, PMS, menopausal issues, diabetes, and other epidemics that affect many American women. High estriol levels are often observed in female athletes, as well as women who follow a vegetarian or macrobiotic diet. Studies on estriol have demonstrated the potential health benefits of high levels. It's important to note, however, that even "normal" estriol levels are not sufficient. Only levels in high or high-normal ranges have health-enhancing effects.

STUDIES ON ESTRIOL

Some of the best evidence we currently have for the positive effects of high-normal estriol levels comes from studies of obese women. With the exception of osteoporosis, obese women suffer from practically every disease known to science far more often than women of normal weight. Research has shown that overweight women are generally low in estriol but very high in estradiol and estrone. A study conducted at Fujita University in Japan illustrates this particularly well. A group of obese women were tested for an entire panel of hormones, including the three primary estrogens. Not surprisingly, their levels of estradiol and estrone were very high, but they were completely deficient in estriol. Not just "most" of the women or "99 percent" of the women were deficient; *every single* woman in the test group had an estriol deficiency and needed supplementation (*Nippon Naibunpi Gakkai Zasshi* v. 72, 1996). These findings are significant for American women, one-third of whom are obese and two-thirds of whom are overweight. The only real solution is lifestyle and dietary modification, but the study shows that estriol supplementation is also an option for preventing the risk of diseases among obese women.

Additional benefits of estriol are especially important for menopausal women. Kathleen Head, a naturopathic doctor, has done extensive research on estriol and menopause. She published an excellent study complete with nearly fifty credible references emphasizing the positive effects and safety of estriol. Head presents evidence—based on various international studies—that estriol helps reduce menopause symptoms, such as hot flashes and vaginal dryness and atrophy, as well as restore healthy vaginal flora and oppose androgen (male hormone) dominance. Additionally, estriol has been shown to lower levels of luteinizing hormone (LH) and follicle-stimulating hormone (FSH), which typically become raised during menopause. Head also discovered that estriol helps support memory and brain function, stabilize mood, build bone, lower blood pressure, lessen the risk of breast cancer, and improve urogenital conditions like incontinence, which can occur in menopausal and postmenopausal women.

There is more research that supports these findings, including studies on urogenital conditions and osteoporosis—an epidemic among elderly women in Western societies (see page 69). The condition does not affect rural Asian women, however, due to their healthy diet and regular physical activity. Osteoporosis can be prevented and managed, but a treatment program that includes diet and lifestyle is necessary. Balancing estriol levels should also be a treatment component, as estriol promotes bone and joint health. This benefit has been demonstrated in studies published in the *Journal of Obstetrics and Gynecological Research* (v. 22, 1996), *Maturitas* (v.1, 1979), *Nippon Sanka Fujinka Gakkai Zasshi* (v. 48, 1996), *International Journal of Gynecology and Obstetrics* (v. 92, 2006), and *Nippon Ronen Igakkai Zasshi* (v. 33, 1996). Estriol therapy is most effective when included in a comprehensive program consisting of diet and lifestyle changes, basic hormone balance, resistance exercise, and nutritional supplements proven to help bone health, like flaxseed oil (see page 120), vitamin D (see page 124), glucosamine (see page 121), and various minerals.

Finally, there are studies showing estriol's positive effects on urinary health, which can decline with aging and result in numerous problems like vaginitis (vaginal infections, such as those caused by yeasts), vaginal atrophy, and urinary tract infections, among others. Doctors have found that estriol supplementation can help reduce urinary tract infections (*New England Journal of Medicine*, v. 329, 1993) and vaginitis (*Turkish Journal of Medical Science*, v. 28, 1998). This is an important discovery, as these infections are common among women, particularly those going through menopause, and can be difficult to treat. The Turkish study used a combination of estriol and acidophilus supplements and was highly successful. This combination of low-dose estriol and acihdophilus was also used in a study conducted two years earlier, where it was successfully used to treat bacterial vaginosis (*Arzneimittelforschung*, v. 46, 1996). There was an 88-percent cure rate, and no other treatment besides estriol was used.

Yet another study conducted at the University of Sassari in Italy and published in the journal *Menopause* (v. 11, 2004) found that estriol supplementation alone can improve overall urogenital health, including incontinence, vaginal atrophy, urinary tract infections, and vaginal infections. No other treatments were used in the study, and the results were impressive. Furthermore, in Basel, Switzerland, doctors directly administered only 0.5 mg of an estriol gel (containing 500 mcg of estriol per dose) to their female patients daily. They reported that "atrophy symptoms were alleviated almost immediately" (*Archives of Gynecology*, v. 239, 1986).

Chinese doctors also had success in treating vaginal atrophy with estriol suppositories (*Zhongguo Linchuang Yaolixue Zazhi*. v. 16, 2000). In Denmark, the same treatment was used for women with urinary incontinence and urgency, dysuria (painful urination), and nocturia (the need to urinate at least two times during the night), and was met with similar success (*British Journal of Gynecology*, v. 107, 2000). The same results were achieved in the Netherlands, where doctors applied the treatment to cases of general urogenital atrophy (*European Journal of Obstetrics and Gynecology*, v. 71, 1997). All of this success makes one wonder why medical doctors in the United States are not using estriol as well.

It is interesting to note that estriol cream (containing 0.1 to 0.3 percent pure estriol) also acts as a skin enhancer, and has been shown to reduce scarring. Usually, only surgical procedures can diminish scars, and these methods are expensive and of limited effectiveness. At University Hospital in Finland, women with acne scars were treated with topical estriol cream, resulting in overall thickening of the skin, including the elastic fibers on their faces, and significantly reduced scarring (*Annales Chirurgiae et Gynaecologiae*, v. 76, 1987). These results are remarkable from a medical standpoint. Similarly, doctors at the University of Hautlink in Vienna successfully demonstrated that raising blood estriol levels in women with acne improved their condition (*Zeitschrift für Hautkrankheiten*, v. 58, 1983). In addition, a group of studies published in the *International Journal of Dermatology* (v. 34, 1995) and the *Archives of Dermatological Research* (v. 256, 1976) showed the effectiveness of estriol for both men and women with acne. One particular study reported the successful treatment of atrophic acne scars, which were dramatically reduced in only ninety days with 0.3 percent estriol cream.

Yet, while the benefits of estriol for the skin have been known for over thirty years, the medical community in the United States has yet to adopt it as a treatment. By contrast, the research on estradiol and estrone is not only overwhelming, but also often unnecessary and repetitious. The effects of estriol should be more thoroughly explored, especially for various diseases and medical conditions. The more we learn about this basic hormone, the more benefits we will find for women who are deficient.

DOSAGE GUIDELINES AND CONSIDERATIONS

As mentioned in Chapter 2, estriol is not manufactured or sold in the United States. US pharmacies do not carry the hormone, and they are unable to special-order the oral tablets from the countries where estriol is readily available. Although some of the studies mentioned above have used oral estriol, it is better to take sublingual and transdermal estriol, which is more potent. One milligram of sublingual estriol is equal to ten milligrams of oral estriol, which causes unwanted metabolites. Doctors will see even more dramatic and impressive results of estriol treatment when they begin to use it in its proper sublingual and transdermal forms.

Since most conventional doctors in the United States are unfamiliar with estriol, they probably will not be able to give you much information about it. However, it is possible to obtain a prescription for transdermal or sublingual estriol through a doctor and have it filled by a compounding pharmacy, as they are not available through regular pharmacies. If you decide to use transdermal estriol, use a 2-ounce jar or bottle that is certified by the USP (US Pharmacopeial Convention). You can find 2-ounce containers of estriol (150 mg) online for only about twenty dollars. Also, do not take homeopathic estriol products, which are also ineffective since they barely contain estriol. Instead, obtain a 2-ounce jar or bottle, which contains about 150 mg of estriol, and apply 0.5 g to the skin each day. Always use transdermal estriol on thin skin, such as that on your neck, abdomen, and inner wrists. Vaginal gels and suppositories are inconvenient and unnecessary. DMSO solutions are 99-percent absorbable but not FDA-approved.

Using sublingual drops is the best way to supplement with estriol, since about 99 percent of the hormones are absorbed into the bloodstream. By comparison, only about 20 percent of estriol creams are absorbed by the blood. When using sublingual drops, which are available through a compounding pharmacist with a prescription, take 0.5 mg (one drop) per day, which is a total of 500 mcg of estriol daily. Make sure that the product you use is a vegetable-oil blend.

Wholesale estriol is very inexpensive, sold at about two dollars per 1 g (1,000 mg). However, compounding pharmacists may charge you fifty dollars for fifty cents' worth of estriol. While online pharmacies outside of the United States do not sell estriol products, it's possible to find quality American-made products for about twenty dollars online.

CONCLUSION

Despite scientific research, estriol remains almost completely unknown in the United States, where it is essentially the "forgotten" estrogen. Considering its demonstrated potential to improve women's hormone balance and overall health, estriol should be embraced by the mainstream medical community. Women should have more options when it comes to balancing their hormones in a natural way, and using estriol is one way to avoid potentially dangerous pharmaceutical drugs. The next chapter explores another vitally important hormone in which many menopausal women are deficient: progesterone.

4. Natural Progesterone

When using hormone supplements, you should always use bioidentical forms in doses that restore and maintain youthful hormone levels. The purpose of taking bioidentical hormones is to achieve natural hormone balance and have the ideal levels typical in young adulthood. This is one of the Seven Steps to Natural Health (see page 143) and a key to life extension. Youthful hormone levels promote optimal health and longevity, and *progesterone*—an essential hormone that regulates the female cycle—plays an important role. Although most forms of hormone therapy use harmful synthetic *analogs* (chemical alterations) of progesterone, there are natural forms available that offer health benefits without increasing health risks. This chapter provides a general overview of progesterone, as well as its most widely prescribed synthetic analogs, and offers recommendations for using its bioidentical forms in a safe and effective manner.

WHAT IS PROGESTERONE?

Progesterone, a female hormone produced in the ovaries and adrenal glands, is needed to maintain proper menstruation and support pregnancy. In pregnant women, who have much higher progesterone levels than non-pregnant women, the placenta also produces progesterone. When used as part of hormone replacement therapy for menopausal women, progesterone offsets the potentially negative effects of excess estrogen (estradiol and estrone), which can thicken uterine lining, stimulate breast tissue, increase blood pressure and blood clotting, cause salt and fluid retention (edema), promote inflammation, accelerate aging, increase body fat and weight gain, and support the growth of tumors, cysts, cancers, and other malignancies. Excess estradiol and estrone can also exacerbate the symptoms of both arthritis and menopause. In contrast, progesterone maintains the uterine lining (endometrium), promotes the maturation of breast cells, normalizes blood sugar and blood clotting, lowers blood pressure, and inhibits the development of cancer, tumors, cysts, and other malignancies. Additionally, the hormone builds bone cells (osteoblasts), boosts immunity, relieves inflammation, reduces the symptoms of menopause, aging, and arthritis.

In excess, estrogens have very toxic effects, while progesterone has protective effects. In moderation, estradiol and estrone are important for good health, but they can pose a danger when levels become high or when there is not enough progesterone to balance them, which is also known as *estrogen dominance*. Progesterone deficiency, a characteristic of menopause, can also be due to factors such as poor nutrition (especially diets high in sugar), insufficient exercise, chronic stress, and disorders like insulin resistance. For this reason, progesterone therapy has become more common among menopausal women, and women of childbearing age alike. Unfortunately, women are hardly ever prescribed natural progesterone. Instead, they are given harmful synthetic analogs called progestins.

NATURAL PROGESTERONE VS. PROGESTINS

Nearly all commonly used supplements and hormones are *synthetic,* which means they are made in a laboratory rather than extracted from a biological organism. For example, despite what vitamin manufacturers may tell you, synthetic vitamin C is always used in supplements because it far less expensive than natural vitamin C. Bioidentical hormones, even though they are the chemical and biological equivalents of natural hormones, are also synthesized. Bioidentical progesterone—along with estrogen, testosterone, pregnenolone, melatonin, DHEA, and various other hormones—are not obtained from cadavers or dead animals, but rather synthesized from soy sterols and other natural bases, such as yam diosgenin.

The most commonly prescribed form of progesterone is neither natural nor bioidentical. Instead, unnatural analogs of real progesterone are contained in most progesterone products, such as birth control pills, as well as used in traditional hormone therapies for menopause. These unnatural analogs are known as *progestins.* Surprisingly, medical doctors and other health professionals often refer to progestins as "progesterone," which is completely inaccurate and misleading to patients. Taken orally, progestins are both chemically and biologically different from progesterone. They are completely unnatural, possess none of the wonderful benefits of progesterone, and have many serious side effects. By law, these side effects must be listed on the package insert of every progestin product. Five specific side effects, eight contraindications, ten adverse reactions, and five major health risks are specified. That's twenty-eight compelling reasons not to take them. Among the many side effects and risks are liver malignancy, cystitis (inflammation of the bladder), depression, fatigue, headache, nervousness, insomnia, dizziness, epilepsy, asthma, cardio-pulmonary aggravation, and further reduced levels of progesterone. Add to this list fluid retention, possible birth defects, blood clots, breast cancer, menstrual irregularities, skin problems, and weight gain, and you are forced to wonder why anyone in their right mind would even consider taking a drug so dangerous—or, better yet, why doctors would prescribe them.

Progestins should never be prescribed, as they have no valid use or benefit. This applies to birth control pills, nearly all of which contain progestins. The most commonly prescribed patented progestin is medroxyprogesterone, or Provera, which can cause the side effects listed above. Obviously, the main reason that toxic drugs like progestins are so heavily marketed and sold to unsuspecting women instead of inexpensive, non-prescription, natural, bioidentical progesterone is profit. There is no other reason to give women costly, dangerous, and unnatural prescription analogs with a long list of serious side effects and no real benefits. Unlike progestins such as Provera, natural progesterone cannot be patented for profit.

TESTING YOUR PROGESTERONE LEVEL

It is rare to have high progesterone levels, especially after menopause. Therefore, it is not necessary for you to test your progesterone level if you are over forty years of age. Women who are still having periods should be assured that their estrogen levels are sufficient; otherwise, they wouldn't be menstruating. Unlike other hormones, progesterone cannot be measured with a saliva test, since it is a fat-soluble hormone. Measuring your progesterone may require a visit to a doctor's office or lab so that a health-care professional can administer a blood-serum (not plasma) test. This distinction is important; since progesterone is fat-soluble, a blood-serum test is the only way it can be measured. It is also very important to note that progesterone testing must be done at specific times during your cycle if you are still menstruating, so you must keep track of your menstrual status.

Keep in mind that blood tests performed by medical doctors require an office visit and can be expensive. In addition, many doctors, including gynecologists and endocrinologists (hormone specialists), are generally not well versed in natural hormone replacement therapy. You must have your free (unbound) levels of hormones tested and then take the necessary bioidentical hormones in proper doses. (A "free" hormone is not attached to carrier proteins, making it bioavailable.) Remember, you should not take oral testosterone, progesterone, estriol, estrone, or estradiol. These hormones must be used transdermally or sublingually. You should be responsible for your own health rather than depend on a doctor. You can achieve natural hormone balance on your own, since bioidentical progesterone creams are readily available on the Internet and do not require prescriptions. In addition, progesterone supplements have a wide latitude of safety. After all, levels are about ten times higher during pregnancy, when progesterone production increases from about 20 mg per day to about 400 mg per day. Natural progesterone is very safe and nontoxic, and there are no known side effects. Use Internet labs such as www.walkinclinic.com.

TAKING NATURAL PROGESTERONE

Like bioidentical estriol, natural progesterone—when taken in normal doses—has no known side effects or contraindications. However, progesterone is not absorbed when taken orally. The liver breaks it down into unwanted byproducts and metabolites, so very little progesterone is actually absorbed into your blood. But since regular pharmacies carry only oral supplements, doctors often prescribe these ineffective substances in high doses. Do not take progesterone injections or suppositories (anal or vaginal), which are totally unnecessary and impractical. And while progesterone can be administered via nasal spray, this method has not yet been approved by the FDA. Sublingual drops (10 mg of a vegetable-oil blend daily) work, but they are not available without a prescription.

Transdermal progesterone creams are by far the most effective and convenient way to use the hormone, as well as the safest and least expensive. With the exception of DMSO transdermal solutions, progesterone cream is available over the counter, which means that you do not need a prescription. Transdermal progesterone is also absorbed well (about one-third), since it readily penetrates the skin and can enter the bloodstream directly, bypassing the liver.

Be sure to use a quality product. Some dishonest hormone supplement manufacturers used to put plain yam extract into progesterone creams, telling women that the substance was the "biological precursor" to real progesterone, and that the body would "convert" it into the natural hormone. Obviously, science does not support these claims. Similarly, homeopathic progesterone products barely contain any of the hormone and are thus ineffective. Products must clearly state how many milligrams of USP progesterone they contain, so be sure to read the label. If a cream or gel does not specify its amount of progesterone, do not buy it. Quality products generally contain about 800 to 1,000 mg in a 2-ounce container, which works out to about 400 to 500 mg per ounce. These usually cost about ten dollars. Progesterone in bulk will usually cost you about fifty cents per gram, so there's no need to pay more than this amount.

If you have a specific medical problem, like fibrocystic breast disease or endometriosis, you can apply progesterone cream directly to the area that is affected. Always apply the cream to soft thin tissue, not thick areas of skin. Breasts, abdomen, inner thighs, and inner wrists are all soft, thin tissue that progesterone penetrates well. If you apply this to thick skin, like stomach or arms, the progesterone will basically just penetrate the skin and tend to stay in the fat cells rather than enter the bloodstream.

Dosages of progesterone vary for pre- and postmenopausal women. If you still get your period, use progesterone cream from day 12 of your cycle to day 26. (Day 1 is the first day of your period.) This way, you will follow the natural cyclical pattern, as progesterone is naturally released by the ovarian follicles during this time. Applying one-half teaspoon to the areas of your body that have thin skin equates to about 30 mg total progesterone on your skin, which means about 10 mg will be absorbed into your bloodstream. During perimenopause, when periods are irregular, it is more difficult to follow this pattern. Just do the best you can and make sure you use the cream for fourteen out of twenty-eight calendar days. After menopause, use one-quarter teaspoon per day for two weeks of every calendar month. This will put about 5 mg total progesterone in your body, which is a sufficient amount. Always use progesterone for the same two weeks every month. A 2-ounce jar should last you more than two months.

You will benefit greatly if you continue to use progesterone for the rest of your life. Remember, you still have one-third of your life left after menopause. Make it a healthy, happy, and fulfilling time. Also, there is no need to use amounts larger than those specified here. In general, when it comes to hormones, more is not better. Your goal is a natural balance of estrogens and progesterone, not excessive levels of any hormone, no matter how beneficial.

It is crucial to use natural hormones in natural ways and in normal physiological amounts to maintain youthful levels. Youthful hormone levels help us stay in the best of health and live as long as possible. Progesterone is very safe and nontoxic, especially in the dosage amounts mentioned above. There are many benefits of progesterone supplementation, and more are being discovered. There are quite a number of studies proving that transdermal progesterone creams are effectively absorbed into the blood and can have dramatic beneficial effects. More studies are being done all the time to show that natural progesterone can be of great benefit to women in ways we haven't yet discovered.

CONCLUSION

Progesterone is a very beneficial hormone, but it is only one part of the endocrine picture. Its benefits are greatest when it is supported by all the other hormones. It is important to realize that our endocrine system, which is made up of ductless glands that secrete our hormones, is a united and synergistic system. Hormones—including progesterone and the three estrogens—work in concert as a team, and they work best when they are at youthful levels. You now know how essential estriol and progesterone are to the body, and why you should take them in their natural form to support hormone balance and boost your health, especially as you approach and go through menopause. It's important to correct both high and low hormone levels, since unbalanced hormones contribute to many health problems prevalent among menopausal women. In the next chapter, you'll read more about your other basic hormones, what they are, and how to test and balance them to achieve optimum health. DHEA, pregnenolone, melatonin, testosterone, T3, T4, growth hormone, and even LH, FSH, and prolactin are all vital hormones. Always keep in mind that these hormones must work together synergistically, which requires balanced, youthful levels.

5. Other Basic Hormones

You are already familiar with the primary female sex hormones, their functions, and how to maintain balanced levels. But there are other hormones that must also be kept within optimal ranges in order for you to achieve total hormone balance. Cortisol, DHEA, growth hormone (GH), insulin, melatonin, pregnenolone, prolactin, follicle-stimulating hormone (FSH), luteinizing hormone (LH), testosterone, and your thymic and thyroid hormones are also involved in basic bodily functions that keep you healthy. This chapter explains the key roles that these hormones play in your health and how to balance your levels naturally.

CORTISOL

Cortisol is considered the "stress hormone" because its primary action is controlling your body's stress response. It also helps regulate glucose metabolism, insulin release, inflammatory response, immunity, and blood pressure, among other vital biological functions. Cortisol levels change throughout the day and can vary dramatically depending on a number of factors, such as physical or emotional stress, vigorous physical activity, injury, and infection.

Chronically high levels of cortisol can lead to heart disease and many other health problems, so it's important that these levels are kept as low as possible most of the time. The best way to do this is by making lifestyle changes that reduce stress and learning stress management techniques. Maintaining a healthy diet and exercising regularly are also essential. Yet, cortisol deficiency is also unhealthy and can indicate an underlying medical condition, such as adrenal insufficiency. Very low cortisol levels can be raised with a bioidentical form of cortisol, like hydrocortisone (Cortef), at the exact time they are low. However, this is not easy to coordinate. Do not bother measuring your cortisol, as it requires a saliva profile that can be found only by testing your levels four times over a twelve-hour period, or every three hours.

DHEA

Dehydroepiandrosterone, better known as DHEA, is the precursor to male and female sex hormones or androgens and estrogens. Countless clinical studies have shown the importance of this adrenal hormone to longevity, immunity, memory, blood pressure, and stress management, as well as the prevention of conditions like obesity, high cholesterol, diabetes, and some forms of cancer. DHEA also plays a role in sexual function and fulfillment, reproductive health, bone density (especially after menopause), and overall sense of well-being.

Levels of DHEA begin to fall around the age of twenty and are generally very low by the age of sixty (see the chart below). Low levels can be treated naturally by taking bioidentical DHEA supplements orally in doses of 12.5 mg (or one-half of a 25-mg tablet) per day. Women usually do not require a larger dose unless they are elderly or ill. You should strive to reach and maintain a DHEA level typical of a healthy thirty-year-old. There is no

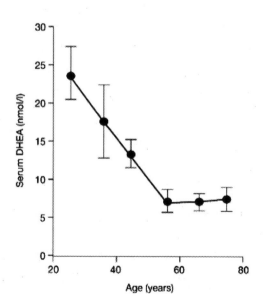

Change in DHEA Levels By Age

universal normal range, but based on ZRT Laboratory's reference ranges, a level of 3.0 nanograms per milliliter (ng/mL) is ideal.

Because DHEA is a very powerful hormone, do not take it without testing your levels beforehand to make sure you have a deficiency. Always use the supplements responsibly by following the instructions on the label and the advice of your health-care provider. An excess of DHEA is also harmful, but there are no supplements currently available for lowering it. If your level is too high, diet and lifestyle change is the only effective natural remedy.

GROWTH HORMONE (GH)

Produced by the pituitary gland, *growth hormone* (GH) is responsible for maintaining your body's tissues and organs. Low levels, which generally occur in middle and old age (see the chart below), can decrease bone density and muscle mass. Unlike other hormones discussed in this chapter, a GH test requires four blood draws over a twelve-hour period (9:00 AM, 1:00 PM, 5:00 PM, 9:00 PM), which must be done at a lab. Insulin-like growth factor (IGF-1) is not an indicator of growth hormone levels—although conventional wisdom says otherwise—so do not try to determine your GH level based on this lab value. Some supplements on the market claim to raise growth hormone but are actually ineffective, so don't give in to persuasive false advertising schemes. Sublingual GH in DSMO solutions are effective, but such prescriptions are not legal in the United States. You can temporarily increase your GH levels by taking 1 g

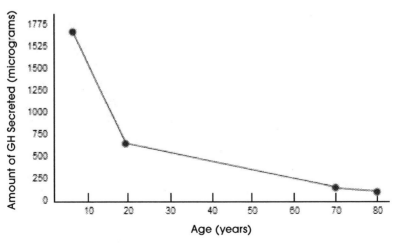

Growth Hormone Decline

of L-glutamine twice a day, in the morning and in the evening. The only way to raise your levels with supplements in the long-term is with injections of recombinant, or synthesized, rHGH. Since it's a long 191-amino acid chain, this substance is expensive to make; a one-month supply (30 IU or 10 mg) will cost you over two hundred dollars, plus the cost of office visits. If you can afford it and are over fifty years of age, take 1 IU per day. Otherwise, you can keep your GH level elevated by following a healthy diet, exercising, breaking bad habits, and focusing on total natural hormone balance.

INSULIN

Insulin is a hormone secreted by the pancreas that enables the body to utilize and store glucose taken in through food. People with diabetes do not have sufficient insulin. In type 1 diabetes, the pancreas is unable to produce insulin. In type 2 diabetes, cells do not respond to normal insulin levels properly. Another form of insulin dysfunction is insulin resistance, the precursor to type 2 diabetes. This has become an epidemic in the United States due to our excessive intake of sugar, refined foods, and saturated fats, as well as lack of exercise, mineral deficiencies, and high obesity rates. This condition occurs when insulin becomes ineffective at lowering blood sugar, resulting in excess insulin to which the cells are unable to respond. Instead of testing your insulin levels directly, you should have a glucose tolerance test (GTT), which evaluates how your body uses and responds to insulin. The GTT is the gold standard for diagnosing insulin and blood sugar dysfunction, but it is very underutilized. See Chapter 12 (page 91) for more information about insulin and insulin testing.

MELATONIN

Sometimes called the "aging clock" hormone, the main function of *melatonin* is to regulate the body's internal clock, which determines when you sleep and wake up. Like DHEA, melatonin is vital for longevity. It influences every cell in your body, acts as a powerful antioxidant, and according to some studies in humans, it may have anti-cancer properties. Melatonin has been the subject of clinical studies and several good books, and there is some evidence that it can strengthen the immune system, alleviate sleep problems associated with menopause, and fight conditions like breast cancer, insomnia, and fibromyalgia. Yet, its importance continues to be underestimated.

As you can see on the chart on page 33, melatonin levels peak during your childhood and slowly decline throughout your life. Levels are normally the lowest during the daylight hours and increase at nighttime to promote sleep. Women tend to have lower levels than men, so those who are over fifty should take about 1.5 mg (one-half of a 3-mg tablet) of melatonin every night. Do not take melatonin during the day, as it causes drowsiness. Testing is optional, but if you want to monitor your level, you can take a saliva test at 3:00 AM.

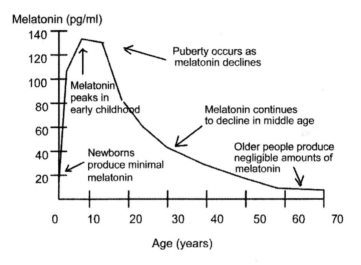

Decline in Melatonin Levels

PREGNENOLONE

As the precursor to all other sex hormones, *pregnenolone* has been called the "grandmother hormone." Like estriol, it is a forgotten hormone, and little research has been done on it. Medical doctors, including endocrinologists, rarely acknowledge or talk about the importance of pregnenolone, which is involved in brain metabolism and has been promoted for memory enhancement. It has also been reported to help conditions like depression, fatigue, arthritis, menopause, and PMS.

As you can see on the chart on page 34, pregnenolone levels fall considerably around the age of thirty-five and then decline at a gradual rate (*Journal of Endocrinology and Metabolism*, v. 82, 1997). Women over forty can take 25 mg of natural (bioidentical) pregnenolone per day, and men, 50 mg per day. Pregnenolone must be taken orally, as it cannot be dissolved and is poorly absorbed through the skin. The hormone is particularly beneficial when used along with phosphatidylserine (PS) and acetyl-L-carnitine (see pages 122 and 118). Again, you want to achieve the level you had at about

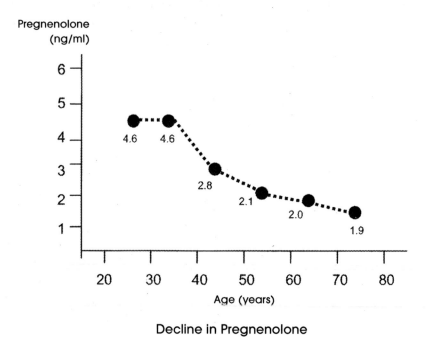

Decline in Pregnenolone

the age of thirty. Although saliva tests are not available for pregnenolone, you can order an inexpensive at-home blood testing kit through www.walkin clinic.com.

PROLACTIN, FSH, AND LH

Often grouped together, prolactin, FSH, and LH are secreted by the pituitary gland and regulate reproductive functions. *Prolactin* is responsible for stimulating milk production and breast development, and is most frequently measured to determine the cause of infertility, irregular or absent periods, decreased sex drive, and other related problems. *Follicle-stimulating hormone*, or FSH, does exactly what its name suggests: it stimulates the ovarian follicle, which includes the egg and surrounding fluid, and the hormones needed to support pregnancy. Like prolactin, it is tested to check for conditions like infertility and menstrual problems. And finally, *luteinizing hormone*, or LH, triggers *ovulation*, the stage of the menstrual cycle when the uterus is prepared to support possible implantation of a fertilized egg. If any of these three levels is too high or too low, the only way to normalize them is by changing your diet and other aspects of your lifestyle in order to support hormone balance. Remember that FSH and LH levels vary dramatically throughout the month in women who are still having periods. Unless you have a condition or suspect that you have a problem, testing these three hormones is optional but can be done through an online laboratory.

TESTOSTERONE

Generally thought of as an exclusively male hormone, *testosterone* is actually produced in women in much smaller amounts by the adrenal glands and the ovaries. Women have only about one-tenth as much testosterone as men; while men produce about 6 to 8 mg per day, women are estimated to produce between 300 and 600 mcg. Testosterone is vital to many biological processes in both males and females, especially the building, maintenance, and repair of your bones. It also influences sexual desire and fulfillment, energy, and muscle strength.

Both high and low levels of testosterone can cause problems, so regular testing is advised. If your level is high, a healthy diet and lifestyle is the only way to normalize it. This rule applies to all androgens. To treat low levels of testosterone, which usually occur in women during menopause (see the chart below), you can take bioidentical testosterone either trans-

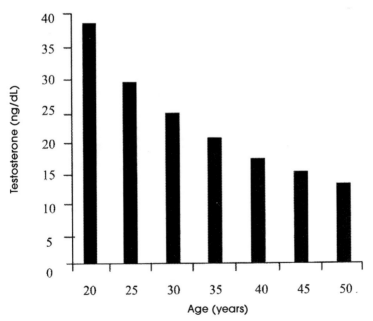

Average Testosterone Levels in Premenopausal Women
(*International Journal of Fertility*, v. 47, 2002)

dermally or sublingually. Start with a dose of 150 mcg (0.15 mg). You can get this amount by applying one-fourth of a gram (750 mcg) to the skin, which will allow 150 mcg to be absorbed. Natural testosterone products usually contain 300 mg of the hormone and are sold in 100-g units, which should last you for at least one year. The most effective method, though, is to use sublingual drops made from a vegetable-oil solution and that contain 200 mcg of testosterone enanthate (150 mcg of actual testosterone) per drop. This substance can be obtained through a compounding pharmacist. Take one drop daily. A 10-mL suspension in vegetable oil is the equivalent of about 320 drops and 64 mg of testosterone enanthate, which should be about an eleven-month supply. It's important that you take testosterone only transdermally or sublingually. Do not take oral or injectable testosterone, and be aware that testosterone nasal sprays have not yet been approved by the FDA.

Test your testosterone levels regularly using a saliva testing kit, and continue to take bioidentical supplements until you achieve a youthful level typical of a healthy thirty-year-old. Based on ZRT Laboratory's reference ranges, women should have a level of 40 nanograms per deciliter (ng/dL), and men, 100 ng/dL. You do not have to measure your androstenedione, as levels usually parallel testosterone levels.

THYMIC HORMONES

The thymus, located in the upper chest, produces four hormones that are essential for immune function: *thymic factor* (TF), *thymosin*, *thymic humoral factor* (THF), and *thymopoein*. Working together, these hormones support the maturation of T-cells and B-cells—lymphocytes that aid immunity. However, the thymus gland atrophies as you age and eventually no longer produces these hormones. Currently, there is no way to replace the hormones or regenerate the thymus, but research is underway. Finding a natural supplement to support thymus activity will go a long way towards achieving better health and a longer life.

THYROID HORMONES

The thyroid gland produces hormones that are needed throughout life. In children, these hormones are essential for growth and development, while their primary functions in adults are metabolism regulation and energy production. The two most important hormone levels you should know and test regularly are T3 (*triiodothyronine*) and T4 (*thyroxine*). Make sure you test your *free* T3 and T4 separately, not *total* T3 and T4. "Free," or unbound, hormones are unattached to carrier proteins and biologically active. High levels of thyroid hormones (overactive thyroid, or *hyperthyroidism*) are far less common than low levels (underactive thyroid, or *hypothyroidism*) among American adults, especially those over forty. This is particularly true for T4 levels.

Effectively raising a low thyroid level with natural hormones can be done very safely, easily, and inexpensively. If you are deficient, you can take any generic brand of cynomel or levothyroxine, which are bioidentical to the hormones naturally produced by the body. Name brands like Cytomel (T3) and Synthroid (T4) are expensive. Do not use products like Armour— thyroid gland extract from pigs—which contain T3 and T4 in a ratio of one to four. This will increase the levels of both hormones, even if you are deficient in only one.

It's crucial for you to maintain free T3 and T4 levels that fall in the middle of the normal range. Do not be led into thinking that any result within the normal range is ideal; both low-normal and high-normal values can indicate a problem. You can test your levels without a doctor through www.healthcheckusa.com.

HOME HORMONE TESTING

It's very important for you to test the levels of all the basic hormones discussed in this chapter, as well as the three estrogens and progesterone. You can get blood tests done by a doctor, but these are usually invasive, expensive, and require an office visit. Moreover, many doctors do not distinguish between hormones that are bound to carrier proteins and those that are freely circulating, which can skew a blood or saliva analysis. When certain proteins in the blood called sex hormone-binding globulins (SHBGs) attach themselves to sex hormones, the hormones become biologically unavailable. Therefore, including bound hormones in a blood or saliva analysis does not paint a true picture of your hormone levels. For example, about 98 percent of testosterone is bound to proteins, yet doctors often measure bound and total testosterone. Lastly, doctors often do not emphasize the distinction between natural and synthetic hormones. As you already know, many doctors use the terms "progesterone" and "progestins" interchangeably, which confuses and misleads patients.

Fortunately, there is an easier, less expensive way that you can test your hormone levels without ever having to step inside of a doctor's office. Saliva testing kits, which are meant to be used in the convenience and comfort of your own home, are available in stores, as well as through online retailers and labs. Saliva-based hormone tests have been administered in clinics for decades, but only recently have they been made available to the general public. This significant medical breakthrough means that anyone can now monitor the levels of their basic hormones at low cost and without the supervision of a doctor.

These saliva kits are easy to use and usually provide clear instructions for self-administering the test, as well as a chart of reference ranges according to sex and age so that you can easily compare your levels to normal, abnormal, and optimal values. Always test your levels at the same time every morning, and do not brush your teeth beforehand, as this will render your results invalid. Also remember that estrogen and progesterone levels must be tested at specific times during the menstrual cycle, which are usually indicated in the testing instructions. After menopause, levels can be tested at any time during the month. Testing kits typically come with a plastic test tube in which you can place your sample and mail it to a lab for analysis. Most laboratories use sophisticated radioimmunoassay (RIA) technology and quickly return your results. You can also use an Internet lab such as www.walkinclinic.com.

CONCLUSION

In general, hormone levels are not measured unless you have a medical condition or symptoms that may indicate a medical condition. This means that maintaining hormone balance and having your levels tested is mainly up to you. *You* must be proactive and take control of this key element in your health; you cannot depend solely on medical professionals. Fortunately, home-testing kits are readily available, and safe, easy, and convenient to use. They can prove to be a vital tool in normalizing your hormone levels and keeping them within optimal ranges. Blood tests can also be ordered through online laboratories that have blood draw centers in various states. Also keep in mind that many natural hormone supplements can be legally obtained over-the-counter or on the Internet without a prescription under US Code 21 (section 331). Just be sure that you do adequate research and choose products from reputable manufacturers that fit the guidelines described in this chapter. As you learn more and more about the importance of the endocrine system, you will understand why balancing your basic hormones is essential to your physical, mental, and emotional health.

6. Premenstrual Syndrome

Medical writings about the occurrence of physical and psychological changes in women leading up to the onset of their periods date back as far as 2,000 years ago. In fact, Hippocrates, the "father of Western medicine," wrote about this condition, which is now referred to as *premenstrual syndrome,* or PMS. The most common symptoms of this syndrome, which affects an estimated two-thirds of American women, include emotional instability, tension, headaches, and irritability. PMS is an epidemic, plain and simple, but it is a very unnecessary one. While most Western women have resigned themselves to this monthly suffering as though it is inevitable, PMS is rarely experienced by women in non-Western countries, especially poor agrarian societies.

Premenstrual syndrome is a complex condition with multiple causes, including diet, hormone imbalance, and a multitude of biological, psychological, and social factors. There is no single or universal cause that can be consistently identified. The only way to deal with such a complicated problem is with a total lifestyle program that includes diet, exercise, supplements, hormone balancing, fasting, and eliminating bad habits and prescription drugs. This chapter is designed to help you eliminate this unpleasant and needless condition with a natural approach that also guides you to optimal health.

WHAT IS PMS?

Premenstrual syndrome refers to a group of symptoms that most women experience in the seven to ten days leading up to their period (menses), which is also called the *luteal phase* of the menstrual cycle. Common symptoms include:

- Abdominal bloating and/or cramps

- Anxiety

- Changes in appetite, including food cravings

- Constipation

- Depression

- Diarrhea

- Fatigue

- Fluid retention, which can lead to minor weight gain

- Headache

- Irritability

- Insomnia

- Joint and/or muscle pain

- Mood swings

- Poor concentration

Most women do not have all of these symptoms and will experience them with varying levels of severity. Symptoms usually increase in intensity as menses approaches, and then cease once it begins or shortly after it starts. There is a very strong hormonal component in this process, but it is not yet completely understood.

Although PMS does not have a single cause, studies have shown that diet plays a central role. A study from the University of Colorado (*Journal of Reproductive Medicine*, v. 32, 1987) looked at the dietary intake of women who suffered PMS symptoms. The doctors found that compared to the average intake of adult females, the women in the study consumed 62 percent more refined carbohydrates, 79 percent more dairy products, 78 percent more sodium, 52 percent less zinc, 77 percent less magnesium, 53 percent less iron, about 50 percent less fiber, and a staggering 275 percent *more* refined sugar and sweeteners. They also drank more coffee than healthy women, and ate fats and proteins from animal sources rather than vegetable oils. The doctors advised the women to significantly cut down on their consumption of simple sugars, meat, poultry, eggs, and dairy products, while eating more fiber from whole grains and beans. The women's calorie intake was decreased, but the addition of fiber to the diet allowed them to feel hungry less often, which promoted weight loss as well. The doctors also suggested supplementing with a variety of vitamins, nutrients, and minerals, such as those discussed in Chapters 16 and 17 (see pages 117 and 131). This simple regimen resulted in a significant reduction in premenstrual problems. Adding natural hormone supplementation for basic hormone balance would have led to even more dramatic results. This study is absolute proof that poor diet—too much fat, too much sugar, too much protein, too many calories, and too little nutrients—is one of the main causes of PMS. After all, as you may recall, women who eat more fat, especially saturated fat from animal products, have higher blood levels of estrogen than women who get 20 percent or less of their daily calories from fats.

Another study that shows the impact of diet on PMS symptoms was done by the Physicians Committee for Responsible Medicine (PCRM), an organization of doctors, including Neal Barnard and Dean Ornish, that was formed to advocate natural health practices. In their study (*Obstetrics and Gynecology*, v. 95, 2000), women were put on a low-fat vegetarian diet for two menstrual cycles. Simply by changing their diet, these women lost weight, their menstrual cycles improved, PMS symptoms were lessened, and estrogen levels decreased, along many other beneficial effects.

These two studies are examples of medical doctors intelligently recommending natural dietary approaches instead of drugs and surgery. Since their publication, a much wider selection of proven natural supplements and hormones have become available, which will undoubtedly provide even more benefits when used in combination with a low-fat diet.

FOUR TYPES OF PMS

Perhaps the most enlightening study ever published on PMS was conducted by Dr. Guy Abraham in the *Journal of Applied Nutrition* (v. 36, 1984). After extensively assessing its complex set of symptoms, he concluded that there were four basic types of PMS: PMT-A, PMT-H, PMT-C, and PMT-D. The significance of his work has never been surpassed. Abraham took a very complicated issue and refined it into a much more comprehensible framework. The four categories are described in the pages that follow.

PMT-A

Affecting more than two-thirds of American women, PMT-A is the most common type of PMS, and is characterized by mostly psychological and mental symptoms rather than physical symptoms. Anxiety, depression, insomnia, irritability, and generalized nervous tension frequently occur. With PMT-A, there is more estrogen (estradiol and estrone) in the body than progesterone, so achieving hormone balance by using bioidentical progesterone is a good way to treat it. Although it is not addressed in the study, estriol deficiency is another common issue in PMT-A.

PMT-H

This is the second most experienced type of PMS among women in the United States. It is very easy to diagnose, as its symptoms are mostly physical in nature, like abdominal bloating, weight gain, breast tenderness, and edema (water retention) in the face, hands, and feet. Researchers have found that women who experience this type of PMS generally have low levels of *dopamine,* a brain chemical that affects cognitive processes like emotional response and the ability to experience pain and pleasure. A healthy diet and lifestyle is the best way to raise dopamine, not medical injections as is common practice in mainstream medicine.

PMT-C

PMT-C occurs in less than 25 percent of women, and is related to blood sugar metabolism and *prediabetes* (see page 92). Symptoms include increased appetite, cravings for sweets—especially chocolate—and hypoglycemic symptoms, such as headaches, fainting, fatigue, dizziness, palpitations, and trembling. High insulin levels are also common. Women who are affected by this type of PMS should treat the condition as they would diabetes, and eat a diet based on whole grains and vegetables while cutting out fruits, dried fruit, fruit juice, sugar and sugar substitutes, and sweets of any kind. A simple, inexpensive GTT is also vital for monitoring blood sugar and keeping levels under 85 mg/dL.

PMT-D

PMT-D is the least common type of PMS and more difficult to define. It occurs in less than 5 percent of women, usually in combination with PMT-A. PMT-D is characterized by mainly psychological symptoms such as depression, lethargy, sadness, crying, confusion, and a general sense of gloom, hopelessness, and helplessness. A small minority of women may even have suicidal tendencies. Women who experience this type of PMS generally have higher levels of progesterone than estrogen, which is unusual. Therefore, hormone balance is needed, but natural progesterone supplements are not necessary.

The system of PMS categories devised by Abraham clearly highlights the complexity of the condition and the varied ways it can affect women. Because PMS does not have a single cause, it is usually treated in ways that attempt to simply eliminate symptoms rather than address the underlying factors contributing to the condition. In most cases, these treatments only create more problems, as you'll see in the next section.

TREATING PMS

Doctors do not have good answers when it comes to PMS. Moreover, they often make the situation worse by prescribing treatments that simply try to eliminate symptoms while ignoring underlying causes. Commonly prescribed therapies include estrogen supplementation (estradiol and estrone), HRT, synthetic progestins, antidepressants, diuretics, anti-anxiety medication, and other harmful drugs without even administering a basic hormone test in most cases. Some doctors have even gone as far as recommending hysterectomies!

Fortunately, there are some enlightened doctors like Guy Abraham who are aware of the literature on PMS. In the same journal article in which he describes the four categories of PMS, (*Journal of Applied Nutrition*, v. 36, 1984), he proposes treatments for each type. For PMT-A he suggests vitamin and mineral supplements, as well as bioidentical progesterone. He also recommends eating more fiber while cutting out dairy, animal products, and desserts from your diet. For PMT-H, he again suggests taking vitamin and mineral supplements, avoiding prescription drugs, and ending bad habits such as smoking and drinking coffee and alcohol. For PMT-C, he recommends minerals, fatty acids (by taking flaxseed oil), cutting out all sweets, and getting a glucose tolerance test (GTT). PMT-D is much harder to treat, and Dr. Abraham calls for a complete physical examination with comprehensive hormone testing. With this type of PMS, there may be high levels of heavy metals in the blood, which can be treated by taking 3 g of sodium alginate (see page 127) per day for one year. If severe depression or suicidal thoughts are experienced, psychiatric counseling is also needed.

Natural treatments fall into three basic categories discussed in the sections below: hormone balance, supplements, and diet and lifestyle.

Natural Hormone Balance

Researchers have observed low levels of progesterone in women who regularly experience PMS symptoms. For example, a study at the Institute of Endocrinology in Moscow found that women who complained of edema prior to the onset of menses were low in progesterone (*Problem Endokrinol-*

ogy v. 25, 1979). At the Umeå University in Sweden, women who had PMT-A symptoms and gained weight at the end of their periods were also found to have low progesterone levels, as well as high levels of estrogen (*Journal of Steroid Biochemistry*, v. 5, 1974). And at the Institute of Endocrinology in Prague, researchers found that women with PMS symptoms generally had low levels of progesterone in the follicular phase of their cycles (the days following the end of the period), as compared to women who did not experience PMS symptoms (*Hormone and Metabolic Research*, v. 30, 1998).

It is rather amazing, but over seventy years ago, Dr. Leon Israel found that "only" 40 percent of women complained of "premenstrual tension" (*Journal of the American Medical Association*, v. 110, 1938). He identified the main symptoms of the condition as tense irritability, crying, headache, vertigo, insomnia, restlessness, breast pain, nymphomania, dysmenorrhea (menstrual cramps), and stomatitis (oral inflammation). He attributed these symptoms largely to low progesterone levels, which he said could be effectively remedied with injections of natural progesterone. Remember, this was before the invention of synthesized bioidentical progesterone, and the only form available was animal progesterone. At the time, most doctors would "treat" the condition by using dangerous radiation, which destroyed the uterus. This practice led to many other horrible side effects, including cancer. Such facts are never talked about or acknowledged. Fifty years from now, it's likely that no one will speak of the fact that nearly one-third of American women had unnecessary hysterectomies. Dr. Israel, however, treated his female patients with progesterone extracted from animals and was successful. Only now, more than seventy years later, are we finally realizing that his approach was the right one.

Katharina Dalton is another doctor who advocated the use of progesterone. A pioneer in women's health who is still cited today, Dalton worked with over 30,000 women since beginning her research more than half a decade ago. In the 1950s, Dalton also noted that 40 percent of women complained of "premenstrual tension" (*British Medical Journal*, 1953). Compare that number to today's figure, which is 70 percent. Dalton also found that excessive estrogen levels caused water retention, one of the classic signs of PMS. She maintained that "the concept of an abnormally high estradiol/progesterone ratio has much in its support." Note her use of the word *ratio* here, as women can have high estrogen, low progesterone, or both. Dalton reviewed earlier studies from the 1940s in which doctors had successfully treated PMS with injections of natural progesterone. (Again, remember that at the time, it was not possible to synthesize natural progesterone, and transdermal progesterone had not yet been discovered.) She also tested the effectiveness of this method and was successful. In a later study, Dalton reported an 83-percent success rate in treating PMS symptoms using high doses of natural progesterone, which were administered to women during the luteal phase of their cycles (*Canadian Journal of Psychiatry*, v. 30, 1985).

A study from the University of Calgary (*Clinical Investigative Medicine*, v. 20, 1997), which also looked at the effects of progesterone on PMS symptoms, had positive results as well. Researchers gave women oral progesterone during the luteal phase of their cycles and noted that there was good general improvement. Transdermal progesterone surely would have produced better results, as oral progesterone requires very high doses and does not absorb well into the bloodstream.

Yet, other studies have had less positive results. PMS is a complex condition, so its treatment is not as simple as just raising progesterone levels. Although numerous clinical studies have established the key role hormones play in PMS, mainstream medical practice rarely emphasizes the importance of overall hormone balance. Melatonin, for example, is crucial. Doctors at the University of California in La Jolla (*Journal of Biological Rhythms*, v. 12, 1997) showed that women who suffered PMS symptoms leading up to their periods generally had low melatonin levels. They said that their findings "replicate the author's previous observation that nocturnal melatonin concentrations are decreased in PMDD [premenstrual dysphoric disorder, a severe form of PMS characterized by symptoms like depression, irritability, and tension]."

Therefore, progesterone supplementation is not a sufficient treatment for PMS, as low progesterone levels are not always the cause of the symptoms. Total hormone balance is needed, so it's important to test your levels of estrogen (estradiol, estrone, and estriol), progesterone, testosterone, pregnenolone, DHEA, thyroid hormones T3 and T4, and melatonin. Glucose tolerance tests (GTTs) are also helpful, as blood sugar disorders can affect PMS symptoms. It is best to keep your blood sugar under 85 mg/dL.

When progesterone is used to treat PMS, though, unnatural progestins should not be used. A study done by Presbyterian Medical Services in New York (*Comprehensive Therapy*, v. 19, 1993) showed that PMS symptoms actually worsened in women who were given synthetic progestins. As already mentioned, some doctors refer to progestins as "progesterone," which falsely conveys the idea that these drugs are the hormone in its natural form. This simply is not the case. Progestins actually decrease the body's production of biological progesterone, leading to even lower levels in the blood and, therefore, even more unbalanced levels.

Supplements

Some natural health practitioners recommend taking various herbs to relieve PMS symptoms. These include chaste tree, dong quai, blue cohosh, and black cohosh, which requires extra caution. The problem here, though, is that all herbs are *exogenous*, meaning that they do not exist naturally in our bodies and are not taken in through the diet. Moreover, everyone has different biological makeup, so an herb that is beneficial for one person may actually be toxic to another and intensify her symptoms. Even if you find an herb that benefits you, it will become useless to you within six months to a year, as the effects of exogenous substances are only temporary. Instead, take the supplements highlighted in Chapter 16 (see page 117). If you are over forty years of age, you should take all the supplements that are listed. It's especially important for women to take vitamin B_6 (10 mg per day) and folic acid (800 mcg per day).

Do not take birth control pills and avoid prescription drugs, as these only worsen PMS symptoms. Obviously, you will be much better off if you use natural alternatives. Talk to your doctor about stopping medication if your condition can be treated naturally instead. Also, ask about other contraception options, since birth control pills are harmful. Good health is simply not possible if you put synthetic, unnatural, and toxic chemicals into your body. Birth control pills and similar medications bring numerous risks and side effects, and they do not address the underlying cause of the problem.

Diet and Lifestyle

Along with balancing your hormones and taking supplements, what and how you eat makes a huge difference when it comes to PMS. The studies discussed on page 40 clearly show the relationship between diet and PMS symptoms. Keep in mind that women who do not eat a high-calorie diet high in fat and refined foods (such as in non-Western countries) do not experience the PMS symptoms that are so common among women in the United States. American women eat twice the amount of calories they need, as well as five times the amount of fat and twice the amount of protein. They also consume 160 pounds of sugar and sweeteners every year, plus large amounts of food preservatives and chemicals, caffeine, and alcohol. These foods must be significantly reduced or eliminated from the diet in order to relieve PMS symptoms. Because women are sensitive to alcohol, which can upset their reproductive system, intake should be limited. Even one drink per day can contribute to medical problems in some women. Coffee can also make PMS symptoms worse due to its caffeine content, as well as the presence of kahweol and cafestol.

Alleviating PMS is also dependent on general healthy living. Exercise is the most important lifestyle element after diet. Female athletes and women who exercise regularly experience PMS less often than women who are not active. This has been demonstrated in numerous studies, including one published in Finland (*Acta Obstetricia et Gynecologica Scandinavica*, v. 50, 1971). They found that women who participated in sports had far fewer PMS symptoms than women who did not. To relieve PMS symptoms and boost your overall health, you should exercise for thirty minutes a day on most days of the week. You can join a gym and take an aerobics class, work with a fitness professional to learn resistance training, take up dancing, or simply go for a brisk walk. Walking is one of the easiest and most enjoyable forms of exercise.

It's important to eliminate habits that can have a negative impact on PMS and your overall health. Smoking, for example, can aggravate PMS symptoms and is connected to problems like premature menopause, osteoporosis, coronary heart disease, and cancer. One-third of American women smoke cigarettes, which partly explains the prevalence of moderate to severe PMS, as well as the multitude of health problems on the rise. If you follow a diet of natural foods, eliminate alcohol and caffeine, exercise regularly, and stop smoking, you will have a much better chance of being symptom-free every month.

Better food choices, beneficial supplements, natural hormone balance, exercise, weekly fasting, and ending bad habits are all part of a total treatment program that will boost your immunity, energize your metabolism, and raise your overall level of health. This way, you will be able to effectively deal with—and ideally eliminate—the very complex, though not well-understood, causes of PMS.

CONCLUSION

Healthy women simply do not experience PMS before their periods. There is nothing "normal" or inevitable about suffering every menstrual cycle, which is inherently symptom-free and healthy. As this chapter has explained, the unpleasant symptoms women experience every month between puberty and menopause are directly linked to hormone balance, which is significantly influenced by diet and lifestyle factors. PMS may be a diverse, complex condition, but that does not mean it cannot be effectively managed and even eliminated. By eating the right diet, exercising regularly, and using beneficial hormone and nutritional supplements, you will greatly reduce PMS symptoms and ultimately rid your life of this condition.

7. Reproductive and Gynecological Conditions

The reproductive system plays a central role in women's health. It regulates the menstrual cycle, facilitates fertilization and conception, and produces the female sex hormones, which influence nearly every function in a woman's body. Obviously, the reproductive system is hormonally controlled and hormonally sensitive, so many gynecological problems are connected to hormone imbalance. Common gynecological conditions range from infections (vaginitis) and vaginal dryness to more serious medical issues like polycystic ovary syndrome (PCOS). There are also gynecological cancers—such as cervical, ovarian, and uterine cancer—that are affecting more and more women. The risk of these medical conditions increases as you age, so it's crucial that you learn how to prevent and treat them naturally. This chapter focuses on some common diseases affecting the reproductive system, and provides basic guidelines for preventing and treating them naturally.

CANCER

The most potentially serious disease of the reproductive system is cancer, which may arise in the cervix, ovaries, uterus, and more rarely, the vagina. More than 80,000 women in the United States are diagnosed with some form of gynecologic cancer each year. However, because symptoms tend to be nonspecific, many women attribute them to less serious conditions and do not seek treatment right away. Some common signs include abnormal vaginal bleeding, unexplained weight loss, fatigue, persistent bloating, pelvic or abdominal pain, loss of appetite, ongoing indigestion and nausea, and frequent urination.

Women with gynecological cancers often undergo a *hysterectomy* (see page 58), which is the surgical removal of the uterus. This risky procedure should always be a last resort, but it may be needed in cases of cancer. Still, before following through with any cancer treatment or procedure, you must do your research and make sure that you have accurate information. Specifically, you should be aware of a treatment's potential side effects, health risks, and effectiveness for your specific type of cancer. One of the biggest problems with conventional cancer therapy is that many treatments are used even if the chances of them actually working are very small. Be sure to ask your doctor these important questions so that you can make an informed decision about the treatment that is right for you and with which you feel comfortable.

Also keep in mind that cancer treatment is ultimately a personal choice. This means that you have the right to try an alternative approach. Natural treatments for cancer address the *cause* of the disease rather than merely its symptoms, which is often the approach taken in conventional medicine. Female cancers like uterine and ovarian cancer are correlated with high estrogen levels which, as you already know, are caused by factors like obe-

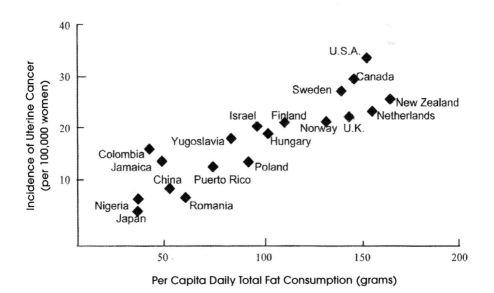

Per Capita Daily Total Fat Consumption (grams)

The Relationship Between Fat Consumption and Uterine Cancer

sity and high-fat diets, as shown in the diagram on page 49. (*Tetrogenesis, Carcinogenesis, and Mutagenesis,* v. 15, 1995). Therefore, a natural way to prevent and help treat the cancer is through diet, supplements, and hormone balance, as well as change to exercising regularly, avoiding unnecessary medications, weekly fasting, and breaking bad habits.

Mina Dobic, the author of *My Beautiful Life,* successfully treated and cured herself of uterine cancer using only natural methods. After being diagnosed, she met several women who had undergone the usual treatments for this type of cancer, such as chemotherapy and radiation. Seeing the permanent damage these conventional treatments had caused, Mina began looking for a natural way to treat herself. She completely changed her diet, eliminating meat, poultry, eggs, dairy products, refined foods, tropical foods, and sweeteners. Mina also started following the traditional Japanese macrobiotic diet, consuming whole grains, vegetables, fruits, and beans. As she states in her book, Mina was free of cancer within one year. This woman, who is no different than you, changed the course of her cancer simply by making better food choices. This inspiring story shows that it is possible to effectively treat and even cure cancer by taking a natural and holistic approach to treatment. And as successful as Mina was, even better results can be achieved by following the less rigid American macrobiotic diet, taking the recommended nutritional supplements (see page 117), fasting regularly (see page 113), and balancing your basic hormones. It's important to take responsibility for your own health and control your own life. Don't let others—including doctors—make your decisions for you.

CERVICAL DYSPLASIA

Cervical dysplasia is a precancerous condition characterized by the abnormal growth of cells on the surface of the cervix. Associated with the human papillomavirus (HPV), this condition is prevalent among females between the ages of twenty-five and thirty-five, and classified from CIN1 (mild) to CIN3 (severe). Women who are most at risk for cervical dysplasia are those who were sexually active at a young age (generally before eighteen), gave birth before sixteen, and have had multiple sexual partners or a history of at least one sexually transmitted disease (STD). Women with HPV, genital warts, or a suppressed immune system due to medication or certain medical conditions are also at high risk, as are those who are smokers or whose mothers took diethylstilbestrol (DES) while pregnant. Cervical dysplasia can lead to cervical cancer, which is frightening, since it often has no symptoms and may not be detected by a routine pelvic exam. Regular pap smears are necessary to test for cervical dysplasia and catch it early.

Cervical dysplasia has become more and more common. It is medically treated with a variety of *allopathic procedures*—therapies that target the symptoms of a condition. A cone biopsy may be performed, in which a cone-shaped piece of cervical tissue is removed. Electrocauterization, a process of destroying tissue using heat conduction, may also be used, as well as cryosurgery, in which extreme cold is used to get rid of the abnormal growth. Laser vaporization, loop electrosurgical excision procedures (LEEP), endocervical curettage, and outright hysterectomies are also often used to treat cervical dysplasia. These invasive procedures can result in permanent damage to the cervix, and even cause infertility, without addressing the cause of the condition in the first place. A less destructive allopathic treatment is topical retinoic acid, but this substance causes side effects that may also be damaging (*Journal American Academy of Dermatology*, v. 14, 1986).

A much more sensible approach to treating cervical dysplasia is following a diet rich in whole, natural foods but low in fat, dairy products, eggs, meat, and poultry. Again, balancing your hormones is crucial. You can use transdermal bioidentical progesterone, applying a cream directly to the abdomen (*International Journal of Cancer*, v. 52, 1992). In addition, take the full array of supplements discussed in Chapter 16 (see page 117) for one year, even if you're under forty years of age. All of these supplements are needed to strengthen your immune system. If you are currently taking birth control pills, estrogen supplements, or other medications, speak to your doctor about stopping these prescriptions. Before resorting to drugs or surgery right away, try a natural approach. It is possible to treat this condition through diet and lifestyle in only a few months without ever having to experience the side effects of conventional treatments.

ENDOMETRIOSIS

Endometriosis occurs when cells from the uterine lining (endometrium) grow in the areas surrounding the uterus, such as the Fallopian tubes, ovaries, bladder, colon, and pelvic cavity. Since these are actual endometrial tissues, they follow the menstrual cycle by swelling with blood and bleeding. This causes internal inflammation and severe pain that becomes worse during menstruation, as well as during the seven to twelve days before the onset of your period. The main complication of endometriosis is infertility. About one-third of infertile women have this condition, which can affect even young women in their teens. But since endometriosis is so closely connected to the menstrual cycle, symptoms generally lessen or disappear altogether after menopause.

Like Alzheimer's disease and AIDS, endometriosis—which was first diagnosed in 1920—was rather uncommon until recently. Today, endometriosis is widespread due to the fact that so many women have high levels of estradiol and estrone, and low levels of progesterone (*Chiba Igaku Zasshi*, v. 69, 1993). Taking bioidentical progesterone can be very helpful for women with endometriosis. Remember, estradiol and estrone promote inflammation, while progesterone mitigates it. It's interesting to note that symptoms of endometriosis are greatly alleviated and even temporarily eliminated during pregnancy, when progesterone levels increase by 1000 percent. However, as mentioned already, women with the condition are often unable to get pregnant or delay becoming pregnant.

Endometriosis is difficult to diagnose because the tiny pieces of tissue outside the uterus often do not show up on tests like x-rays, sonograms, and color Doppler ultrasounds. Usually, only a laparoscopy—the surgical insertion of a tiny medical camera—can detect the condition. It is possible to make a diagnosis based on symptoms and treat the problem with a basic natural approach involving dietary and lifestyle adjustments, along with hormone balance. It's very important to lower your levels of estradiol and estrone, while raising your body's amount of progesterone. (See page 26 for dosage guidelines.) Do not attempt to treat endometriosis with prescription drugs such as dangerous GnRH agonists, birth control pills, danazol, aromatase inhibitors, NSAIDs, and synthetic progestins. You should also not undergo invasive and ineffective procedures like surgery. Even when laparoscopic surgery is partially successful, the tissues simply grow back within two years. Do not consider having a hysterectomy, as this is a drastic and unnecessary procedure for a condition that can usually be treated naturally. (See page 58 for more about hysterectomies.)

FIBROIDS

Fibroids, or *myomas*, are benign (non-cancerous) tumors composed of muscle and fibrous tissue in the uterus that can be very small or grow to the size of a grapefruit. They tend to affect women in their thirties, but generally stop growing when estrogen levels fall after menopause. Uterine fibroids are very common; according to some estimates, about 80 percent of American women develop them at some point in their lives. Black women are more likely to have uterine fibroids than Caucasian women, while a lower percentage of Asian women are affected by the condition. However, since fibroids do not have symptoms, most women are unaware that they have them. Usually, a test such as a simple ultrasound (sonogram) first detects the presence of uterine fibroids, most of which are ultimately benign. It's estimated that malignancy occurs in one out of every two hundred fibroid cases.

Although fibroids do not usually lead to serious medical complications, they can cause the uterus to drop, which, in turn, may lead to urinary incontinence (leakage). Additionally, because women with heavy, painful, and irregular periods are at the greatest risk for fibroid growth, anemia may result due to blood loss. Fibroids do not respond to prescription drugs and are almost always impossible to remove with surgery (myomectomy)— even advanced laser surgery—especially when they develop within the uterus. Hysterectomies are performed when fibroids produce severe symptoms. This is a drastic measure and completely unjustified. Do not get a hysterectomy for fibroids—it simply is not necessary. See page 58 for more information on hysterectomies.

The only way to decrease and eliminate fibroids is through natural methods. Basic hormone balance is vital. Bioidentical progesterone supplements can stop future growth, but in order to shrink existing fibroids, you must lower your estradiol and estrone levels. The most effective way to do this is to follow a low-calorie diet that is low in fat and high in fiber, such as the American macrobiotic diet. Eliminating saturated fats, avoiding alcohol, exercising regularly, and losing weight are also good ways to reduce high estrogen levels. Additionally, women over forty years of age should take the supplements highlighted in Chapter 16 (see page 117), like DIM (200 mg per day) and flaxseed oil (1,000 to 2,000 mg per day), to lower estrogen levels and improve estrogen metabolism. Taking 300 mg of beta-sitosterol daily has also been shown to benefit uterine function (*Biochemical Molecular Biological International*, v. 31, 1993).

Another way to shrink fibroids is through general calorie restriction and a two-week fast, which should be done at a health center. Abstaining from all foods and beverages except water is safe for most people and particularly beneficial for those who are overweight. However, people with diabetes should not fast until they are well, and women who are pregnant or nursing should not fast for longer than one or two days. Short fasts like these are recommended for everyone, regardless of age. You should fast for twenty-four hours—from dinner to dinner—once a week, and do one forty-eight hour fast once a month. Following a low-calorie diet will help your body adjust to fasts more easily so that you do not experience as many side effects, like headaches and irritability. The health benefits of calorie restriction are well documented and have been reported to improve longevity, as well as fight aging and many degenerative diseases. Roy Walford, a medical doctor and professor, has written two great books on calorie restriction as a method of health enhancement and life extension (see Recommended Reading on page 147). See Chapter 15 (page 113) for more information about fasting and calorie restriction.

OVARIAN CYSTS

Small fluid-filled sacs in or on the ovaries, *ovarian cysts* are generally connected to disordered ovulation. They are often asymptomatic but may also cause abdominal pain, lower back pain, painful intercourse and periods, nausea, breast tenderness, difficulty emptying the bladder, weight gain, and pelvic swelling, pressure, or pain. While some ovarian cysts are harmless, symptoms that worsen or include dizziness, faintness, weakness, and rapid breathing signal a more serious problem.

Ovarian cysts, which can be benign or malignant, have become far too common among the Western female population, affecting mainly women in their thirties. The two basic types of cysts are *follicular cysts* and *corpus luteum cysts*. Follicular cysts form when *follicles*—cyst-like structures that normally rupture to release eggs—do not burst open. These cysts are tiny and usually dissolve within ninety days. *Corpus luteum cysts* develop when follicles release the eggs but then reseal themselves, causing fluid to accumulate inside so that the sacs expand and turn into cysts. Corpus luteum cysts tend to be large, but they usually disappear on their own within a few weeks. Three other types of ovarian cysts are:

- **Endometriomas.** Occurring in women with endometriosis (see page 51), these cysts form when uterine tissue attaches to one or both of the ovaries and grows.

- **Cystadenomas.** These develop from ovarian tissue and form on the ovary's outer surface. They may be filled with watery fluid or a mucous-like substance.

- **Dermoid cysts.** This type of cyst contains many different types of cells. They can be large and painful, but they are rarely cancerous.

Polycystic ovarian syndrome (PCOS), which involves multiple ovarian cysts, is discussed in a separate section (see page 56). Ovarian cysts can be detected by a sonogram or color Doppler ultrasound, which will indicate if the growth is malignant or benign. The CA-125 blood test, which is also used to test for ovarian cancer, is popular but unreliable. Cysts are typically treated with surgery or prescription drugs, but these should always be the last resort. The surgical procedure used may either be a laparoscopy, which involves small incisions and local anesthesia, or a laparotomy, which calls for large incisions and general anesthesia. These procedures are risky, and may cause one or both ovaries to lose function. For this reason, cysts should be treated naturally with a healthy diet, nutritional supplements, and bioidentical hormones—a safer, healthier, and more effective approach.

PELVIC INFLAMMATORY DISEASE (PID)

Pelvic inflammatory disease (PID), or salpingitis, is a serious infection of the uterus, ovaries, or Fallopian tubes that can be bacterial, viral, fungal, or parasitic. The infection usually occurs when sexually transmitted bacteria spreads up through the cervix, and into the uterus and upper genital tract. In the United States alone, it's estimated that nearly 1 million women— most of whom are sexually active women under the age of twenty-five— suffer from the condition. Most cases go undiagnosed and untreated. Sexually transmitted diseases are the number one cause of PID, so the more sexual partners you have, the more likely you are to contract it. About half of all PID cases are caused by gonorrhea followed by chlamydia, which is accompanied by milder symptoms. Women who have given birth, had a miscarriage or abortion, douche, use intrauterine devices (IUDs) as contraception, or have a blood infection or lymphatic condition are also at greater risk for PID.

Pelvic inflammatory disease is a dangerous situation that can cause permanent damage to the reproductive system and lead to sterility. About 100,000 women in the United States lose their fertility due to PID every year. Furthermore, scarring resulting from PID can form adhesions to nearby tissues, leading to abscesses and even *necrosis*—the premature death of living tissue. A potentially life-threatening condition known as *ectopic pregnancy* can occur as well, which is when a fertilized egg is planted somewhere outside the uterus. One of the biggest problems with PID is that it is often asymptomatic; two-thirds of women are simply unaware that they have it. However, in some cases, PID causes fever, pelvic pain, painful intercourse, and irregular menstrual bleeding.

In general, pelvic inflammatory disease is very difficult to diagnose, and usually treated with invasive laparoscopy and/or antibiotics. Although transdermal estriol and progesterone creams can help the problem, PID is a chronic condition. The best course of action is prevention, which is possible with the right diet and supplementation, as well as natural hormone balance. Getting tested regularly tested for STDs is the best method of prevention. You should also have all three of your estrogen levels tested and take the appropriate steps to correct an imbalance.

POLYCYSTIC OVARY SYNDROME (PCOS)

As its name indicates, *polycystic ovary syndrome* (PCOS) is characterized by the presence of many small cysts on the outer surface of the ovaries. These cysts form when eggs stay on the surface instead of being released. *Vascular impedance*, or reduced blood flow to the ovaries, is an immediate result. In the long-term, women with PCOS are at higher risk for coronary heart disease, type 2 diabetes, high blood pressure and lipid levels, sleep apnea, uterine cancer, and other diseases, as well as premature death. There is also a high rate of infertility and miscarriage among women with PCOS.

There is more to the disease than just polycystic ovaries. The three cornerstones of the condition are obesity, insulin resistance (the precursor to diabetes), and *androgenicity*—elevated levels of the androgens DHEA, testosterone, and androstenedione. High levels of luteinizing hormone (LH) and prolactin are also common with PCOS, as is low progesterone. In addition to general menstrual problems including menstrual irregularity, women with the condition tend to have one or more of the following symptoms:

- Absent or few periods

- Acne or oily skin

- Depression

- Elevated triglycerides

- Hair loss

- High blood pressure

- Hirsutism, which is characterized by excessive hair growth on the body where women typically have minimal hair

- Low magnesium levels

- Pelvic pain

- Sleep problems

- Unbalanced HDL-to-LDL ("good" and "bad") cholesterol ratio

- Vaginal bleeding

PCOS can be asymptomatic, so it's important to get checked for this condition if you have irregular periods or trouble getting pregnant. Sonograms and color Doppler ultrasounds are safe, inexpensive, and accurate. And since insulin resistance usually occurs with PCOS, it's important that you also get a glucose tolerance test (GTT). It's a good idea to get this test done on a regular basis, since insulin resistance is quickly becoming an epidemic in the United States.

PCOS is treatable through natural means by addressing the three basic cornerstones of the condition: hormone imbalance (androgenicity), insulin resistance, and obesity. You can correct hormone imbalance with bioidentical progesterone cream. Dietary and lifestyle modification will also help lower LH, prolactin, and androgen levels. A total program involving dietary adjustment, nutritional supplements, exercise, and natural hormone balance is necessary for getting rid of extra pounds and treating insulin resistance, which can be reversed by eliminating all desserts, sweets, fruit juices, and foods containing sugar and sugar substitutes from your diet. This includes maple syrup, honey, and any other natural sweeteners. Sugar is sugar is sugar.

OTHER GYNECOLOGICAL CONDITIONS

In addition to the medical conditions discussed in this chapter, there are also more minor problems that commonly affect women. Some of these may become more frequent after menopause due to the imbalance of the vaginal bacterial flora. Such problems include:

- *Atrophic vaginitis*, or dryness due to thinning of the vaginal walls and decreased lubrication
- Genital warts
- *Lichen sclerosus*, a skin condition characterized by white patches on the vulva
- Sexually transmitted diseases, such as herpes
- *Trichomoniasis*, a common STD caused by a protozoa that often leads to vaginitis
- Vaginal dryness
- Vaginal mucous or discharge
- Vaginitis (vaginal infection)
- *Vulvodynia*, or itching, burning, and pain in the vulva
- Yeast infections (thrush)

Fortunately, these ailments are usually treatable. For vaginitis (regular or atrophic), try 1-percent zinc pyrithione, an antibacterial agent that is available as a cream or spray. Vaginal mucous and discharge is often caused by birth control pills or estrogen supplements, so the best solution is to speak to your doctor about stopping these medications. Do not take antibiotics, which are normally prescribed for this condition but address the symptom rather than the cause. Antibiotics also further upset the balance of beneficial vaginal flora. Vaginal mucous can be greatly alleviated by removing dairy products from your diet, as lactose promotes mucous formation in the body. A healthy diet and lifestyle is also essential to reduce vaginal dryness, since emollients are not effective for the condition.

For overall gynecological health, you should follow a healthy diet, take the recommended supplements (see page 117), and use natural (bioidentical) progesterone cream and intravaginal estriol cream. Decades of research have shown the value of intravaginal estriol to treat general vaginal atrophy that comes along with aging and menopause (*Maturitas* v. 3, 1981). This can be obtained only through a compounding pharmacist. Be sure to have your estriol level tested before taking hormone supplements. You may also consider using herbal or acidophilus-based douches, but they should be used only once a week at most, as more frequent use will further upset the natural balance of flora in your vagina. In place of douching, try mixing six capsules of potent acidophilus (at least 6 billion colony-forming units per capsule) in water and inserting it into your vagina while lying down with your feet positioned above your head. There are other safe and effective ways to treat gynecological problems using natural methods. If you suffer from one or more of these medical issues, you should seek the advice of a natural health practitioner.

THE TRUTH ABOUT HYSTERECTOMY

As you already know, in the United States, mainstream medicine is procedure-driven and dominated by allopathic treatments. As a result, surgery—hysterectomy in particular—has become a billion-dollar industry. The United States has the highest rate of hysterectomy in the industrialized world, with an estimated 600,000 procedures performed annually. After cesarean section, hysterectomy—the full or partial removal of the uterus—is the second most common surgery among American women, one-third of whom will have a hysterectomy by the time they reach the age of sixty. Women in the United States are four times more likely to get a hysterectomy than women in Europe, New Zealand, and Australia, and studies have shown that in the majority of cases—as much as 90 percent—the procedure is not medically necessary. Moreover, the majority of American women who undergo hysterectomies are not elderly, as is commonly believed, but rather in their early to mid-forties. This means that each year, the lives of hundreds of thousands of young, generally healthy women are needlessly put at risk.

Contrary to popular belief, cancer and other life-threatening conditions account for only 10 percent of hysterectomies. The most common reasons for the operation include fibroids (see page 52), endometriosis (see page 51), heavy bleeding, polyps (small benign growths in the uterus), chronic pelvic pain, pelvic infections, and uterine prolapse—a condition in which the uterus slides from its normal position into the vaginal area. These situations hardly ever require surgical intervention, as there are plenty of alternative approaches that are safer, less extreme, and more effective. For example, fibroids—the number one reason for hysterectomy—and endometriosis can be treated with lifestyle change and bioidentical hormone therapy. Uterine prolapse can be treated with simple surgical procedures.

Most people are also unaware of the wide range of physical, psychological, and emotional side effects women endure as a result of hysterectomy. According to a study conducted by the HERS (Hysterectomy Educational Resources and Services) Foundation, the most common side effects experienced by women after undergoing a hysterectomy include:

- Personality changes (79 percent)
- Irritability (79 percent)
- Loss of energy (78 percent)
- Fatigue (77 percent)
- Loss of sexual desire (75 percent)
- Memory loss (67 percent)

- Insomnia (61 percent)
- Joint pain (60 percent)
- Hot flashes (57 percent)
- Anxiety (57 percent)
- Achy muscles (55 percent)
- Suicidal thoughts (53 percent)
- Weight gain (52 percent)

And the list doesn't end there. Other reported side effects include hearing loss, sciatica, painful sex, constipation, headache, vaginal dryness, vertigo, edema, visual problems, fibromyalgia, heart palpitations, panic attack, urinary incontinence, carpal tunnel syndrome, and bladder infections. Other problems that may result are arthritis, hair loss, osteoporosis, sinus problems, high or low blood pressure, high or low blood sugar, sexual dysfunction, and many others. The operation itself can cause urinary tract infections, hemorrhaging, ruptured or infection incisions, abnormal blood clotting, internal organ damage, and even heart attack. Plus, there are long-term consequences, including increased risk of osteoporosis and heart disease. According to the famous Framingham Study, hysterectomy may triple the likelihood of heart disease occurrence, especially in women who are forty years of age or younger. Women who are still getting their periods at the time of the operation will go through menopause at a younger age, if not immediately.

Perhaps the most serious consequence of hysterectomy, which Dr. John Lee points out in his book, *What Your Doctor May Not Tell You About Menopause,* is the loss of full ovary function. Since removal of the uterus cuts off the ovaries' blood supply, there is really no such thing as a hysterectomy that "preserves the ovaries." Many doctors either do not realize this fact, or fail to understand the vital role the uterus and ovaries play in not just reproductive functions, but a woman's whole body. In his book, Dr. Lee quotes a doctor speaking to the American College of Obstetrics and Gynecology in 1971 as saying, "...after the last planned pregnancy, the uterus becomes a useless, symptom-producing, potentially cancer-bearing organ and therefore should be removed." Lee's book also contains a quote from an official of the Harvard School of Public Health who said in 1979, "If a woman is thirty-five or forty years old and has an organ that is disease prone and of little or no further use, it might as well be removed." These statements reflect an outdated, inaccurate view of the female body that, sadly, many doctors continue to have.

If your doctor recommends a hysterectomy, obtain a second opinion. Find a health-care provider who understands the risks involved in the surgery, and who will help you search for hysterectomy alternatives if the procedure can be avoided. A hysterectomy is life-changing, so it's important to explore all options before resorting to the operation. Make sure you have the right information about your condition and the treatments available. You should also read Dr. John Lee's books, as well the books on hysterectomy listed under Recommended Reading on page 147. Remember that most gynecological conditions can be prevented and treated with lifestyle modification, a diet of whole natural foods, supplements to support core nutrition, and hormone management.

It's ideal to take a natural approach to health whenever possible. However, you may feel that a hysterectomy is necessary if your condition is life-threatening or unmanageable. If that's the case, do not be alarmed—you do not have to be another statistic. It's still possible for you to avoid many debilitating side effects and health issues associated with hysterectomy. You can also achieve the balanced hormonal profile of a healthy young woman very easily and inexpensively. Be sure to monitor your hormone levels, especially estradiol, estrone, estriol, testosterone, DHEA, T3, and T4 using a saliva test or testing offered by online labs. If you are low in any of these hormones, supplement with bioidentical hormones; if you have high levels, adjust your diet and lifestyle according to the guidelines presented in this book. Women over forty years of age may want to supplement with bioidentical pregnenolone and melatonin as well, and women of all ages can use progesterone cream to boost levels. It's also important to control your blood sugar, cholesterol, and triglycerides counts to prevent medical conditions that may complicate your post-surgery health management. Remember that natural hormone balance combined with a whole grain-based diet, proven nutritional supplements, weekly fasting, and regular exercise can bring about immense change in your well-being and dramatically raise your quality of life.

CONCLUSION

Although the female reproductive system is sensitive and subject to a variety of problems—especially after menopause—your gynecological health is still within your control. Many of the most common ailments, from cervical dysplasia to vaginitis, are linked to hormone imbalance, particularly high estrogen levels. By keeping your hormones balanced and taking a natural approach to your health, you can avoid serious gynecological disorders and diseases that affect thousands of women every year. Also be sure to have regular pap smears, which can detect abnormalities that other medical tests cannot. But do not rely on medical testing when it comes to your health. Prevention, not detection, is your best protection.

8. Breast Disease

As you already know, your basic hormones play a central role in your health. Natural hormone balance is the key to effectively preventing and treating conditions that commonly affect women, including adverse menopausal symptoms, osteoporosis, and heart problems. This is especially true for breast disease, which—as research has shown—is very hormonally sensitive, and directly correlated with high estrogen and low progesterone, particularly among menopausal women. This chapter explores the relationship between hormones and various types of breast disease, explaining how you can prevent cysts, benign tumors, and even breast cancer by taking a natural approach to your health.

HORMONES AND BREAST DISEASE

Your breasts are very strongly influenced by your sex hormones. This is especially true during puberty, pregnancy, and menopause. Estrogen, particularly estradiol and estrone, cause cells to reproduce and spread, which can lead to excessive tissue growth. Cell proliferation and abnormal growth of tissues is usually the first step in the development of breast cancer and other malignancies.

The three most common breast-related problems in women are cysts, tumors, and cancer. A *cyst* is a fluid-filled sac within the breast that can vary in size and texture. Breast cysts are prevalent among women in their thirties and forties, but they tend to disappear on their own after menopause. While there are various causes of cysts, excess estrogen is a contributing factor. A *tumor*, which can be either benign (non-cancerous) or malignant (cancerous), is a dense mass of tissue that grows in an abnormal way. It takes two to sixteen years for breast tumors to grow large enough to be detected during examination. Benign tumors tend to be oval or round, while malignant tumors have an irregular shape. According to recent statistics, breast cancer is the most commonly diagnosed cancer among women besides non-melanoma skin cancer in the United States. The risk of breast cancer increases with age, so older women are particularly vulnerable—especially those who have too much or too little of certain hormones.

As mentioned in Chapter 2, there is a direct relationship between estrogen therapy and breast cancer. A study from Harvard Medical School (*Journal of the National Cancer Institute*, v. 90, 1998) concluded that "data in conjunction with past epidemiological and animal studies provide strong evidence for a casual relationship between postmenopausal estrogen levels and the risk of breast cancer." The report also stated that estrogen and progestins may promote the proliferation of cancerous cells, leading to a higher rate of breast cancer among women who take hormones. In addition, women who take birth control pills tend to have more breast problems than those who do not because of the toxic synthetic ethinyl estradiol contained in these medications. Providing additional proof for the link between hormones and breast disease is that women who have had ovariectomies or hysterectomies—the removal of the ovaries and the uterus, respectively—have less breast cancer due to lower estrogen levels. Excessively high levels of androgens, such as DHEA and testosterone, are also correlated with breast disease, especially breast cancer.

Progesterone, on the other hand, slows and moderates the growth of breast cells and facilitates their maturation, which is why very low levels of progesterone can also lead to breast problems. For example, *anovulatory* women have more breast problems than women with regular menstrual cycles, since their bodies do not produce progesterone (*New England Journal of Medicine*, v. 293, 1975). International research has continually demonstrated that women with low progesterone levels have a much higher risk of breast cancer. They also have ten times the normal rate of death from malignant neoplasms (cancerous growths), and three times the normal rate of death from all causes (*American Journal of Epidemiology*, v. 114, 1981). Other studies have found that women with low progesterone levels suffer more frequently from every possible breast disorder, including *mastitis* (breast infection), *mastodynia* (breast pain), cysts, fibrocystic breasts, and nodularity (*Obstetrics and Gynecology*, v. 54, 1979). Furthermore, studies show that the ratio between estrogen and progesterone is a factor in breast health. Women whose levels of estradiol and estrone are in the high or high-normal range, but who have low levels of progesterone, are prime candidates for abnormal breast cell growth due to an unbalanced ratio. More specifically, there are studies of postmenopausal women with breast cancer showing high estrogen and low progesterone levels (*Pharmacy Science* v. 8, 1995).

All of this data shows how important it is to maintain youthful levels of your basic hormones, particularly when it comes to breast health. It also demonstrates the harmful effects of hormone therapy and birth control pills, which increase your risk of breast cancer. Remember, there are other methods of birth control like tubal ligation, which is safe and even reversible.

THE IMPACT OF DIET ON BREAST HEALTH

In the United States and many European countries, women have a one in eight chance of getting breast cancer in their lifetime. According to Dr. Robert Kradjian, the incidence of breast cancer among women in industrialized countries is about 600 percent higher than among women in agrarian societies. Approximately 85 percent of breast cancer cases occur after the age of forty-five, when progesterone levels fall severely and the estrogen-to-progesterone ratio becomes dramatically unbalanced.

Epidemic-like rates of breast cancer have occurred mainly in affluent Western countries with a predominantly Caucasian population. Despite endless propaganda about how we are supposedly winning the "war on cancer," the death rate among American women still has not improved. In fact, it gets worse every year. The reason has nothing to do with genetics or family medical history, as only 6 percent of identical twins both get breast cancer, and only 2.5 percent of women with breast cancer have family members who have also had the disease (*Journal of the American Medical Association*, 1993).

So then what's to blame? The main culprit is the Western diet, which is high in saturated and trans fats. Fat intake is the number one reason for high breast cancer rates in the United States and Europe. The chart on page 66, which is based on the fat intake (in grams) of various female populations, clearly shows the relationship between fat consumption and breast cancer. In the thirteen countries with the highest cancer rates, women get about 40 percent of their fat calories from animal sources (*Cancer Research*, v. 45, 1985). By contrast, in many Asian and African countries, only about 10 to 15 percent of daily calories are from fat—most of which comes from vegetable oils—and breast cancer rates are much lower. For example, only 1 in every 120 Kenyan women has breast cancer, since they obviously do not have the luxury of eating a high-fat diet. Migration studies also point to the relationship between the Western diet and breast cancer. The rate of breast cancer dramatically increases when non-Western women immigrate to the United States and adopt the cultural diet.

Saturated fats from animal sources—the dangers of which have been discussed in previous chapters—is not the only thing to blame. Always remember that high fat intake translates to high estrogen levels, which, in turn, lead to high breast cancer rates. Ignore the health professionals who say that "early detection is your best protection," and remember that *prevention* is your best protection. You can prevent breast cancer by eliminating red meat, poultry, eggs, milk, and other dairy products (including yogurt) from your diet. Milk products contain lactose, an allergen, as well as casein, a substance that has cancer-promoting properties. According to a study published in the *British Journal of Cancer* (v. 61, 1990), the rate of lymphoma is several times higher among women who drink milk than those who do not. A study published in the *American Journal of Epidemiology* (v. 130, 1989) showed a higher rate of ovarian cancer among female milk drinkers as well. There are numerous studies supporting these findings. Today, there are plenty of tasty substitutes for dairy-based milk, cheese, cream cheese, and yogurt, so there is no reason for you to consume dairy products. Caffeine and alcohol are also correlated with breast disease, so eliminate them from your diet, as even small amounts can have a negative impact on your breast health.

Protection against breast cancer and other cancers can be achieved simply by following a diet that contains less than 20-percent fat. The fats you do eat should come from vegetable oils such as corn oil, safflower oil, olive oil, sesame oil, sunflower oil, and flaxseed oil. You may have heard about studies denying that there is a relationship between fat intake and breast cancer, such as Harvard's Nurses' Health Study. However, their report is misleading because the diet followed for the study contained 32-percent fat, which is only slightly lower than the usual 42 percent. Therefore, the disparity was insignificant and did not make any real difference. The critical level for fat intake is less than 20 percent, preferably down to 15 percent. Ideally, only 10 percent of your daily calories should come from fat, which is normal in many cultures around the world.

PREVENTING BREAST CANCER

The biggest lie told about female cancers is that "early detection is your best protection." Organizations that promote the fallacy of "early detection" mislead innocent women into thinking that this is more important that preventing the disease in the first place. *Prevention* is your best protection. Prevention is the answer to breast cancer, but it can be achieved only with a low-sugar, low-fat diet and general healthy living.

Researchers at the European Institute of Oncology in Milan conducted a very interesting study involving 5,517 women to find out the specific factors correlated with high breast cancer rates in Italy. They discovered that alcohol consumption, low intake of beta carotene (see page 118), low intake of vitamin E (see page 124), and lack of exercise were especially important. They stressed that these four factors are very easy to modify, and that doing so would prevent at least one-third of the breast cancer cases in Italy. The study also highlighted the positive effects of nutritional supplements, which are very beneficial when it comes to preventing breast cancer and maintaining breast health. Supplements are also effective for preventing prostate cancer, which, interestingly, is the male equivalent of breast cancer in females. In addition to vitamin E and beta carotene—a pigmented compound in mostly fruits and vegetables—beta-sitosterol (see page 119) has been shown to have benefits for breast cancer, as well as other forms of cancer like prostate and colon cancer, when taken in doses of 300 mg per day. Diindolylmethane, or DIM (see page 119), in doses of 200 mg per day is also effective for lowering estrogen levels and improving estrogen metabolism so that the more potent estrogens in your body are converted into less potent forms. CoQ_{10} (see page 119) is very beneficial for breast health as well, which was demonstrated in a study conducted at the University of Texas (*Biochemical and Biophysical Research Communications*, v. 3, 1994). In the study, doses of CoQ_{10} were given to women who were receiving no other

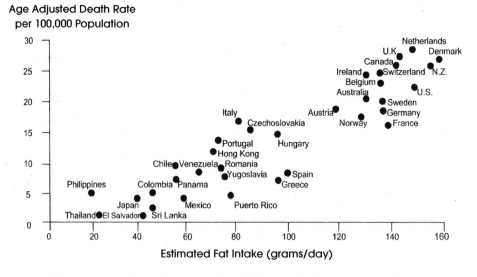

International Breast Cancer Death Rates Related to Fat Intake

treatments for breast cancer. Remarkably, all patients showed improvement, and some even had their tumors disappear within only three months. This important supplement should be taken in doses of 100 mg per day. Flaxseed oil (see page 120) supplements should be taken as well to help regulate estrogen levels. A 1,000-mg softgel capsule or one-half teaspoon of bulk flax seed oil is an appropriate daily dose. See Chapter 16 (page 117) for information on additional supplements you should take for both disease prevention and optimal wellness.

There are also bioidentical hormone supplements you can take for breast health in addition to progesterone and estriol. The hormone melatonin (see page 32) is vital for protection against cancer in general, but it is especially effective against breast and prostate cancer. At the Medical University of Lodz in Poland, doctors determined that "preliminary results of use of melatonin in the treatment of cancer patients suggest a possible therapeutic role for melatonin in human malignancy" (*International Journal of Thymology*, v. 4, 1996). German doctors at the University of Tübingen also studied the relationship between melatonin and cancer, finding that "a progressive decline of pineal melatonin secretion was observed parallel to the growth of primary breast and prostate cancer indicating substitution therapy to be promising" (*Wiener Klinische Wochenschrift*, V. 109, 1997) And at the Cancer Registry in Norway studies of 15,000 women found that those with the lowest levels of melatonin had the highest rates of breast cancer (*British Journal of Cancer* v. 84, 2001).

DHEA is another hormone that is important for preventing and treating cancer, particularly breast cancer. At the famous Johns Hopkins University in Baltimore, Maryland, researchers found a strong relationship between low DHEA levels and breast cancer (*Cancer Research* v. 52, 1992). More specifically, they found that the average DHEA level among women with cancer was 10 percent lower than the study's control group—women who did not have cancer. However, there was also a high rate of cancer among women with excessive levels of DHEA. In other words, DHEA is a double-edged sword; both high and low levels are correlated with higher cancer rates in women. Therefore, you must measure your DHEA level before taking hormone supplements and continue to measure it regularly, which goes for all the other androgens as well.

Taking nutritional and hormone supplements—especially in combination with diet, a natural exercise, and an overall healthy lifestyle—is the best natural way to protect against cancer. However, it is commonly believed that regular mammograms are sufficient protection because they offer "early detection." Again, early detection is a fallacy; prevention is always the answer. Mammograms are risky and can actually stimulate malignancy because they expose you to radiation. There are much safer, effective ways to test for breast cancer, including MRIs, sonograms, and Doppler radar. Avoid unnecessary medical testing and choose safe alternatives over high-risk procedures.

CONCLUSION

Considering the epidemic-like rates of breast cancer and other breast diseases, it may seem like it's just a matter of time until you experience this firsthand, if you haven't already. But you do not have to be a statistic. There are plenty of natural ways to prevent breast disease, such as restricting your fat intake, exercising regularly, taking beneficial supplements, and balancing your hormones. To put it simply, there is no reason at all for you to ever suffer from a breast condition. Whether you are young or old, it is possible for you to take control of your health and avoid these diseases by adopting healthy lifestyle practices. Remember, prevention, not detection, is your best defense against disease.

9. Osteoporosis

In general, people tend to think of bones as being rigid and dead, much like the anatomical model skeletons found in laboratories. But quite the opposite is true. Bones are alive, dynamic, and constantly generating new cells to replace old ones. About every three months, your body forms small, spongy *trabecular bones,* and about every twelve years, you develop dense, compact *cortical bones.* Simply put, you are always growing new bones, which remain healthy throughout your life provided you give them the right nutrients, keep them strong with exercise, and perhaps most importantly, maintain balanced hormone levels.

Bone health is particularly crucial for women, who tend to lose more bone density than men as they age. Osteoporosis, the most commonly diagnosed bone disease, is prevalent among menopausal women, particularly in the United States, due to factors such as hormone imbalance, poor diet, and lack of strength-building exercise. It is possible to reverse osteoporosis and rebuild lost bone cells, as well as prevent osteoporosis from developing in the first place. But in order to do so, you must adopt a total lifestyle program of dietary modification, nutritional supplements, exercise, and bioidentical hormones. This chapter provides basic facts about osteoporosis and dispels common myths about how it arises. It also tells you how to avoid the debilitating condition using only natural methods, ensuring that your bones remain strong throughout your life.

WHAT IS OSTEOPOROSIS?

Osteoporosis is the gradual thinning of bone tissue and bone density over a period of time, resulting in brittle bones that fracture easily. The condition occurs when the body no longer forms enough new bone, when too much old bone is reabsorbed by the body, or both. In young people, new bone is produced by the body more quickly than old bone is broken down, thereby increasing bone mass. Typically, people have the most bone mass when they are in their early twenties. Through the natural process of aging, however, the body begins to lose bone mass more quickly than new bone is made, which is why older adults—especially women—are at higher risk for developing osteoporosis than younger adults.

The risk of bone loss and osteoporosis is increased by factors such as high intake of protein and saturated fat, excessive sugar, salt and caffeine consumption, mineral deficiency, soda consumption (which contains an excessive amount of sugar, caffeine, and phosphoric acid), alcohol or tobacco use, lack of exercise, and chronic stress. Each of these factors is common to the typical American lifestyle, which explains why rates of osteoporosis are so high among older women in the United States. Because hormones also play a significant role in maintaining healthy bones, unbalanced levels can contribute to bone deterioration. Women who undergo a hysterectomy are at higher risk for developing osteoporosis, since female reproductive organs are one of the primary sources of hormone production. Estrogen controls *osteoclasts*—the cells responsible for removing dead cells from the bones—while *osteoblasts*, which build bone tissue, are regulated by progesterone and androgens (male hormones) like DHEA, testosterone, and androstenedione. Estriol, the "good estrogen," is also influential in this process. This is well documented by science, but the mainstream medical community has yet to incorporate this knowledge into its standard practices.

Osteoporosis is an epidemic among women in the Western world. But this is not the case for other parts of the world, especially non-industrialized countries in Africa, Asia, and South America, where people suffer from bone and joint disease at far lower rates. This proves that bone diseases like osteoporosis are caused by factors that can and should be controlled. However, there are a couple popular myths about the cause of the disease that have prevented it from being treated properly.

THE TRUTH ABOUT OSTEOPOROSIS

Osteoporosis, like any other illness, is not some mysterious "accident" that cannot be understood. It's widely believed that the condition is linked to calcium deficiency, which is not at all the case. Women (as well as men) in Western countries consume more calcium than any other population in the world due to excessive intake of dairy products. Yet this same group of women also has the highest rate of osteoporosis and other bone diseases, as well as hip fractures and arthritis. Half of all Caucasian women over the age of fifty have serious bone loss, which begins around the age of thirty-five.

This simply was not common in the United States 100 years ago, and the main culprit for the dramatic increase of osteoporosis is poor diet.

Nearly all of the calcium in the Western diet comes from dairy products. The USDA claims that you need at least 1,000 mg of calcium per day for good health. This is ridiculous, since eating large amounts of high-allergenic foods like milk and cheese is basically the only way you can meet this requirement. It also does not explain how people in other cultures, particularly Asia, do not include any dairy in their diet at all and yet have lower rates of osteoporosis and other bone diseases. And finally, the body cannot absorb calcium unless it also has sufficient amounts of magnesium, boron, strontium, silicon, vitamin D, vitamin K, and other bone-building nutrients. In other words, consuming significant amounts of calcium is useless when it comes to bone health if you do not have adequate levels of the nutrients that are needed for calcium absorption. Instead, take 250 mg of bioavailable (easily absorbed) calcium per day. That's all you need.

The other prevailing myth about osteoporosis is that it can be caused by estradiol and estrone deficiency, which has led doctors to prescribe estrogen therapy to menopausal women for bone loss. However, taking estrogen supplements—especially horse estrogen—does not build or strengthen bones. Estrogen therapy with estradiol and estrone has no effect, since these two estrogens merely control the cells that remove the dead bone (osteoclasts), while progesterone and androgens stimulate the cells that build new bone (osteoblasts). A 1995 study published in the *New England Journal of Medicine* tracked 9,500 women on estrogen over an eight-year period, and ultimately found that the therapy had zero benefits for bone health, especially with regard to hip fractures—the single most debilitating injury resulting from osteoporosis. Approximately half of the women who suffer a hip fracture never walk again. Estriol, on the other hand, is never prescribed for osteoporosis treatment, even though it has been shown to have positive effects on bone metabolism, as well as powerful bone-building potential.

The fact of the matter is that most American women begin to experience bone loss long before menopause, usually when they are in their mid-thirties—when estrogen levels are at an optimal youthful level. However, they may not experience any negative symptoms for twenty years or more. As a general rule, women lose about 1.5 percent of their bone cells each year in the two decades leading up to menopause. At eighty years old, most women have only about half of the bone mass they had at the age of forty. Imagine having only *half* of the bone strength that you have now. It's frightening to know that you can expect to have only 50 percent of your bone cells at some point in your future.

Neither calcium deficiency nor estrogen deficiency is to blame for osteoporosis. In reality, it is low levels of progesterone, as well as certain male hormones—such as DHEA and testosterone—that very often trigger bone deterioration. As already mentioned, these hormones regulate osteoblasts, the cells responsible for bone formation. Researchers at the University of British Columbia conducted the best review ever published on the subject of progesterone and bone health, entitled, "Progesterone as a Bone-Tropic Hormone" (*Endocrine Reviews*, v. 11, 1990). The study presents overwhelming evidence that progesterone is the bone-building hormone. The late Dr. John Lee, a well-known author of books on natural health for women, supported these findings in his 1991 study, "Is Natural Progesterone the Missing Link in Osteoporosis Prevention and Treatment?" (*Medical Hypothesis*, v. 35, 1991). In his article he states, "The hypothesis that progesterone, not estrogen, is the missing factor [in osteoporosis prevention and treatment] was tested in a clinical setting and was found to be extraordinarily effective in reversing osteoporosis." Yet the scientific evidence has not changed how osteoporosis is treated by most medical doctors.

The role of androgens in bone health, as well as women's health in general, is also often overlooked since they are thought of as exclusively male hormones. However, women need DHEA, testosterone, and androstenedione just as much as men do, but in smaller amounts. A study conducted by scientists at the Indiana School of Medicine observed 231 women between thirty-two and seventy-seven years of age, and found that progesterone, along with DHEA and testosterone, were positively correlated with bone density (*Journal of Endrocrinology*, v. 97, 1996). Specifically, premenopausal women had levels of 0.17 nanograms (ng), while postmenopausal had levels of 0.07 ng.

Along with the other medical conditions mentioned in the previous chapter (see page 62), low progesterone levels can contribute to osteoporosis. Progesterone deficiency in women of childbearing age may be due to *anovulation,* a state in which ovulation fails to occur during the menstrual cycle. Anovulation does not usually have symptoms, so women often do not know that they have it. Thus, you should be proactive and start progesterone supplementation long before menopause, when you are between thirty and forty years of age. (See page 26 in Chapter 4 for dosage guidelines for progesterone supplements.) Blood serum testing will tell you if your body is producing enough progesterone, or if the supplements are effective. However, you can avoid this situation entirely by following a healthy diet, doing resistance exercise, and taking a natural approach to hormone balance.

PREVENTING AND TREATING OSTEOPOROSIS

There are no shortcuts when it comes to preventing and treating osteoporosis. It requires a total program that touches upon every aspect of your lifestyle, including nutrition, eating habits, and exercise. Unfortunately, medication is generally thought to be the answer, even though commonly prescribed drugs for osteoporosis do not work and have never worked. You'll find that no matter what you hear in the media about osteoporosis drugs, taking medication will not help the condition. Every year, a new "miracle drug" for improving bone density is touted by pharmaceutical companies but never lives up to its promises, often making the condition worse. The advertising for such drugs is often persuasive, but do not be fooled by it. Prescription drugs do not cure osteoporosis. You must deal with the causes of bone loss, not just the symptoms.

The most important factor in the prevention and treatment of osteoporosis is diet. You must reduce your intake of animal fats and protein, as well as sugary foods like sweets. These foods acidify the body and upset *acid-alkaline balance*—the ratio between acids and bases in your body. Nearly half (42 percent) of the calories in the typical American diet comes from fats, especially saturated animal fats. The average American also consumes about 160 pounds of sugar every year, which is completely unnecessary and unhealthy. Dairy products, even those that are low-fat or nonfat, should also be avoided due to their lactose and animal protein (especially casein) content. As already mentioned, American and European women consume the most dairy products out of any other female population in the world, and yet have the highest rates of arthritis, osteoporosis, and bone disease. Websites like www.notmilk.com and www.milksucks.com provide additional reasons to stay away from milk and other dairy products. They should be completely eliminated from your life. Also moderate your consumption of salt, as well as alcohol, coffee, and soda.

Vitamin D_3 is the most important substance to take, as the body cannot absorb calcium without it. Science has shown that there are many other benefits to having plenty of vitamin D in your system, but most people are deficient in it, as it cannot be obtained from the diet. Although it is called a "vitamin," vitamin D is actually a hormone found only in tiny amounts in some animal products like eggs. Its production can be stimulated by exposure to the sun, but most people are not in the sun enough to make sufficient amounts, especially during the winter. This is why you should take vitamin D_3—the form of vitamin D that is active in humans—as a supplement in doses of 800 international units (IU) per day. If one tablet contains only 400 IU, take an additional 400 IU. But do not exceed 1,200 IU per day, no matter what you hear or read. See Chapter 16, "Essential Vitamins and Other Nutrients," (page 117) for more about vitamin D_3.

In addition to following these nutritional guidelines, you should engage in resistance exercise to strengthen your bones. *Resistance exercise*, also known as strength training, is exercise that is performed to increase muscle mass and bone strength. One reason that women in non-industrialized countries tend to have strong bones is because manual labor and physical exercise is part of their lifestyle. In contrast, most Western women, particularly in the United States, rarely do strenuous work requiring muscular exertion. The incidence of osteoporosis among obese women, however, is lower due to the fact that their bones must be strong enough to support all the extra weight they carry. An investment of one hour per week for resistance exercise is all it takes to build your strength, stay fit, and keep your bones strong. Swimming is a great exercise, as well as weight training with light free weights. With the help of a fitness professional, you can learn to "superset," or perform one set of exercises after another continually. Set aside just one half hour two or three days per week for some type of resistance exercise, which can be done at a gym or in the comfort of your own home. The combination of a nutritious diet, proven supplements, and strength-building exercise will significantly help you reduce your risk of osteoporosis, as well as provide many other health benefits. A full spectrum of proven supplements is also needed, including glucosamine, flaxseed oil, vitamin D, and a complete mineral supplement. (See Chapters 16 and 17 on pages 117 and 131 for more information on these supplements, as well as dosage guidelines.) This is the best way to prevent and cure bone loss naturally. Please do not resort to pharmaceutical drugs, as they simply do not work.

TESTING FOR BONE LOSS

Regular hormone testing is essential when it comes to monitoring your bone health. The hormones that play a central role in bone growth and development—progesterone, estriol, DHEA, and testosterone—should be measured regularly with a saliva test. This is very important for menopausal women. Remember, you should try to achieve the youthful hormone levels that you enjoyed around the age of thirty, rather than simply maintain a level that is "normal" for older adults. See the chapters on estriol and progesterone (pages 17 and 23) for information about sublingual and transdermal bioidentical hormone treatments, which you will need if you are low on either of these hormones. If you are low in DHEA, you can take 12.5 mg per day. Levels of testosterone and androstenedione are likely to parallel one another, so if they are low, sublingual or transdermal hormones can be used. Women need only about 150 mcg of testosterone in total per day. Do not use the hormone in its oral or injected forms. It is rare for women to have high androgen levels ("androgenicity"), but if this is the case for you, use natural means to lower your level. There is no pharmaceutical drug that can reduce your levels as effectively or as safely as a healthy diet and lifestyle. See Chapter 5 (page 29) for more about supplementing with these hormones.

While hormone testing can be done at home, bone loss must be measured by a physician. To do this, a technique called *dual photon absorptiometry* (DPA) is preferable to *dual energy x-ray absorptiometry* (DEXA). Although both methods are about 97 percent accurate, DEXA uses low-level radiation, while DPA uses photons, or light energy. In general, it is a good idea to avoid radiation whenever possible, so choose DPA.

CONCLUSION

Although bone density declines with age, you can foster bone growth and maintain bone strength even during your postmenopausal years. Contrary to popular belief, neither low estrogen nor calcium deficiency is the cause of osteoporosis among aging women. Rather, it is low levels of progesterone, estriol, and the androgens—particularly DHEA and testosterone—that contribute to bone deterioration, in combination with an unhealthy diet and lack of exercise. The best way to ward off osteoporosis is to balance your hormones naturally through healthy eating, nutritional supplementation, and bioidentical hormone treatment when necessary. Regularly testing your hormone levels before, during, and after menopause will enable you to keep track of your hormone balance, bone health, and general well-being.

10. Arthritis

The leading cause of disability in the United States, some type of joint inflammation affects almost nearly every American over the age of sixty-five. Approximately 50 million adults—most of whom are women—have some type of arthritis, which impacts mobility, quality of life, and even mood. Pharmaceutical drugs commonly prescribed by medical doctors merely attempt to suppress arthritis symptoms without addressing its underlying causes. And despite the endless media hype and advertisements, wonder drugs for arthritis never work and often come with numerous side effects. There are few published studies on natural arthritis treatments, but as you will find out in this chapter, the condition can be easily prevented and alleviated with a healthy diet, active lifestyle, nutritional supplementation, and natural hormone balance.

WHAT IS ARTHRITIS?

Arthritis is the inflammation of one or more joints, usually due to aging, injury, or an autoimmune disorder. When cartilage breaks down, the joints become enflamed, which, in turn, causes the surrounding bones to painfully rub together. There are more than 100 types of arthritis, the most common forms being *osteoarthritis* and *rheumatoid arthritis*. Both of these types are more prevalent among women than men. *Osteoarthritis* is caused by normal wear and tear, while *rheumatoid arthritis* is an autoimmune condition. Symptoms generally include pain, swelling, stiffness, and decreased mobility. Overweight and obese people are at higher risk for arthritis, as excess pounds put more stress on your joints, especially in the knees, hips, and spine. A poor diet and hormone imbalance also promote the condition (see pages 77 and 80).

Medical treatments for arthritis usually focus on relieving symptoms or minimizing damage instead of addressing the actual cause. Common remedies include pharmaceutical drugs like analgesics (painkillers), nonsteroidal anti-inflammatory drugs (NSAIDs), and corticosteroids, as well as injections of drugs directly into the joints. Not only do these treatments produce numerous side effects, but they are also ineffective—they do not cure the disease. A total lifestyle program of dietary modification, exercise, supplements, and natural hormone balance is required to treat the condition effectively.

ARTHRITIS AND YOUR DIET

Many studies have shown that joint inflammation is linked to the foods you eat (*Journal of Clinical and Biological Chemistry*, v. 20, 1996). The worst culprits are saturated fats from animal products, as well as hydrogenated and partially hydrogenated oils (trans fats), which do not exist in nature (*Pharmacology*, v. 51, 1995). In addition to inflammation, these fats contribute to clogged arteries, heart attack, stroke, and altered hormone levels (*British Journal of Nutrition*, v. 61, 1989). In countries where people eat fewer calories and less meat, sugar, and refined foods, the rates of bone and joint problems are much lower (*Nutrition Research*, v. 14, 1994). This is especially true in poor countries. These statistics support the link between a high-fat, high-sugar diet and inflammation.

Vegetables in the nightshade family can also contribute to inflammatory conditions in the body. Studies have shown that joint problems improve when these vegetables are removed from the diet. The nightshade family includes poisonous plants like tobacco, Jimson weed, and deadly nightshade, as well as commonly consumed vegetables like potatoes, tomatoes, eggplant, and peppers. Nightshade vegetables contain a compound called solanine, and tomatoes contain tomatine in addition to solanine. Solanine and tomatine are toxic *alkaloids*—naturally occurring substances that can produce pharmacological effects in humans and animals. A study of hospital patients demonstrated that nightshade vegetables can also have strong allergenic effects (*American Medical News*, January 25, 1999), in turn causing inflammation in the body. You must eliminate or restrict nightshade vegetable intake in order to prevent joint inflammation. Replace potatoes with whole grains, and completely cut out tomatoes, peppers, and eggplant.

It's important to emphasize the role that food allergies play in the relationship between arthritis and diet. Allergens produce inflammation in the body, so eating certain foods to which you are allergic or sensitive can contribute to arthritic conditions (*Inflammation and Drug Therapy Series*, v. 5, 1992). Most people, however, are not aware that they have food allergies, since symptoms can be subtle, delayed, or nonexistent. Therefore, food elimination strategies for identifying allergens are useless. Moreover, tests commonly used to detect food allergies, such as the ALCAT and ELISA tests, are inaccurate and inconsistent. The best thing you can do to prevent an allergic reaction and, therefore, joint inflammation is to eat a low-calorie, plant-based diet low in sugar, fat, and protein, and high in fiber, complex carbohydrates, and other whole natural foods. The whole grain-based macrobiotic diet is ideal, since it is the least allergenic of all diets. Whole grains, beans, and most vegetables are the least allergenic and should be staple foods. Omega-3 fatty acids also have anti-inflammatory properties, so be sure to consume flaxseeds or flaxseed oil, which are the best sources.

In addition to eating *better* food, you should also eat *less* food. The average woman needs only about 1,200 calories per day, but most American women take in twice this amount. Studies have shown that calorie restriction is positively correlated with longer lifespan and better overall health (*Science*, August 1999). Eating two meals per day instead of three is a good way to reduce your calorie intake. You may even try eating only a healthy well-balanced snack in the morning or early afternoon, followed by one nutrient-dense meal later in the day. Fasting on water for one day per week can also produce immediate and dramatic effects. Fasting (see page 113) is one of the most powerful healing techniques, helping to flush toxins out of your body and facilitate weight loss. If you have diabetes or a serious medical condition, speak to a holistic or naturopathic medicine doctor before starting a fast.

EXERCISING YOUR JOINTS

Exercise is usually recommended for managing arthritis, but it is also a key to prevention. Regular physical activity helps protect and support the joints, strengthen the muscles, and increase mobility. In addition to its physical benefits, exercise boosts your mood and improves your overall quality of life. Plus, exercise is essential for weight loss, which reduces the stress on your joints.

An ideal exercise regimen consists of both aerobic and muscle-strengthening exercises. Aerobic activities include walking, running, biking, dancing, and sports such as tennis and basketball. If you have joint pain, it is best to stick to low-impact exercises like walking or swimming in order to prevent pain and injury. You should do some form of aerobic exercise for thirty minutes at least five days a week. Muscle-strengthening (resistance training) exercises—which include weight training, calisthenics, and using resistance bands—are particularly effective for enhancing joint function. You can do resistance training two or three times a week. Finally, remember to stretch before and after exercising in order to improve your flexibility and protect your muscles and joints from injury.

Although exercise is highly beneficial, keep in mind that it can further damage your joints if they are not well lubricated, or if your cartilage has started to break down. If you have arthritis, consider physical therapy or water aerobics, and refrain from exercise until your condition has improved. Any kind of moderate to intense exercise can be harmful if your joints are inflamed, so it's important to be cautious.

SUPPLEMENTS FOR ARTHRITIS RELIEF

There are a number of nutritional supplements that aid in the prevention, management, and treatment of arthritis. Supplements that promote good digestion—such as acidophilus, FOS, and L-glutamine (see pages 118, 120, and 121)—can be beneficial, since inflammation is linked to intestinal health (*Scandinavian Journal of Immunology*, v. 40, 1994). Glucosamine sulfate has been shown to have positive effects on arthritis, but it is effective only when taken in combination with a multivitamin, complete mineral supplement, a source of omega-3s, and if necessary, a natural hormone supplement. Specifically, you should take the recommended daily amounts of all thirteen essential vitamins especially vitamins C, D, E, and K. Also, instead of taking regular vitamin B_{12}, use methylcobalamin, which is its most absorbable form. Make sure you find a mineral supplement that contains calcium, magnesium, boron, copper, manganese, molybdenum, selenium, silica, cesium, chromium, iodine, vanadium, gallium, germanium, cobalt, nickel, zinc, strontium, and tin. All twenty of these basic minerals are vital for healing inflammation. See Chapter 17 (page 131) for more about mineral supplements. Finally, it is better to get your omega-3 fatty acids from flaxseed oil rather than fish oils. An appropriate dose is 1 to 2 g per day. For general wellness, it is a good idea to take all of the supplements recommended in Chapter 16 (see page 117).

Yet some supplements are not effective for treating for arthritis, despite claims to the contrary. There have been no clinical trials of substances like chondroitin and methylsulfonylmethane (MSM), which is an oral form of dimethyl sulfoxide (DMSO)—a substance found in wood pulp. Applying DMSO solution to the areas of your body in which the joints are swollen or stiff will only raise your blood levels of DMSO, which is dangerous, as it is not naturally present in food or in the body. In other words, using DMSO for arthritis is not a natural health practice. Other popular alternative remedies for arthritis—ginger extract, devil's claw, and cetyl myristoleate (CMO), for example—are also not supported by science. Exogenous herbs like curcumin and boswellin are effective only in the short-term; they should not be used for long-term treatment.

THE ROLE OF YOUR HORMONES

Hormone imbalance is a primary cause of joint inflammation. As you know, hormones work together to carry out vital biological functions, and their "teamwork" depends on balance. Testosterone, DHEA, estradiol, estrone, estriol, pregnenolone, melatonin, T3, and T4 are all influential when it comes to maintaining joint health.

The relationship between progesterone and arthritic conditions was first shown in a study published over seventy years ago (*Mayo Clinic Proceedings*, v. 13, 1938) that focused on pregnant women with arthritis. The researchers found that arthritis conditions significantly improved when progesterone levels increased, which occurs during pregnancy. Several studies published since then support this link.

High estradiol and estrone levels also promote inflammatory conditions, while estriol can help diminish them. This explains why Western women—who tend to be high in estradiol and estrone but deficient in estriol—are at higher risk for arthritis than other female populations. DHEA and testosterone are also vital for bone and joint health (*Arthritis and Rheumatism*, v. 40, 1997), as is melatonin (*Zhonngua Yaolixue Tongbao*, v. 10, 1994). While the relationship between pregnenolone and arthritis has not yet been closely studied, the hormone will surely be shown to be effective.

Additionally, it's important to maintain normal (mid-range) levels of the thyroid hormones T3 and T4, as thyroid disease is strongly correlated with rheumatoid arthritis. Remember, not all values that are technically considered "normal" are actually desirable. By maintaining balanced levels of these basic hormones and testing them regularly, you will decrease your chances of developing joint pain and inflammation.

CONCLUSION

Like heart disease, type 2 diabetes, and osteoporosis, arthritis is an increasingly prevalent public health problem in the Western world. It is now the leading cause of disability among adults in the United States, making it difficult for many individuals to engage in everyday life activities and manage other chronic health issues. Women are disproportionately affected by this debilitating condition. Still, it is possible to treat arthritis effectively by following a low-fat and low-sugar diet, exercising regularly, taking nutritional supplements, and naturally balancing your hormones. Remember, when you take control of your health, you can fight and avoid disease.

11. Heart Disease

The leading cause of death worldwide is *heart disease*, also called *cardio-vascular disease*, which is a group of different diseases that affect the heart and/or blood vessels. Every year, all types of heart and artery disease kill more women in the United States than any other disease or illness. Although heart disease is obviously a major health risk, there is plenty you can do to achieve better cardiovascular health, including making better food choices, taking beneficial supplements, avoiding prescription medications, ending bad habits, fasting once a week, exercising regularly, and of course, balancing your hormones. More specifically, you must keep five blood lab values—cholesterol, triglycerides, homocysteine, C-reactive protein (CRP), and uric acid—within their respective low-normal ranges, not simply the average range or even the normal range. The two most important diagnostic factors are triglycerides and cholesterol, which tend to be very high in American men and women alike. This chapter gives you all the information you need to keep your blood levels within optimal ranges using a natural approach, which includes dietary adjustments, basic lifestyle changes, and taking four key supplements—beta glucan, beta-sitosterol, flaxseed oil, and soy isoflavones.

CHOLESTEROL

Cholesterol is a waxy, fatty substance (lipid) found in the blood that is essential for adrenal and sex hormone production, among a variety of other functions. Of all the blood lipids, cholesterol is the most meaningful diagnostic value, which means that your level can tell you the most about your heart health status. The most common cause of high cholesterol is excessive intake of saturated fats, especially animal fats—for example, red meat, poul try, eggs, and dairy products—which constitute 42 percent of the calories in the standard American diet. The worst fats of all are hydrogenated oils, or *trans fatty acids* (trans fats), which do not exist in nature. Trans fats are found in fried foods and many processed food products, including snack foods, condiments, and commercial baked goods. Vegetarians, vegans, and people who consume seafood as their only "animal product" tend to have healthy cholesterol levels. After all, plants do not contain cholesterol, and the cholesterol found in fish and other seafood does not raise your levels when eaten in moderation.

Due in large part to this high-fat diet, the average cholesterol level among American adults, both male and female, is between 225 and 250 milligrams per deciliter (mg/dL), which is very high. By contrast, the average cholesterol level is 150 mg/dL among adult populations in Asian countries, which is ideal, as shown by the famous Framingham study and many others. The chart below, which reflects the findings of a 1995 study published in *BMJ*, shows a sharp increase in mortality due to high cholesterol when levels climb above about 7.5 mmol/L (which is equal to about 289 mg/dL). The lowest mortality rate is found among women who have cholesterol levels of about 3.4 to 4 mmol/L, or between 135 and 150 mg/dL.

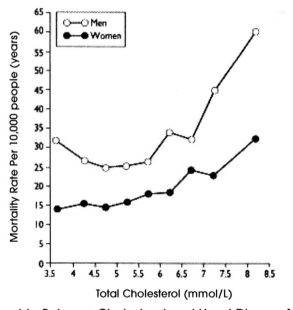

Relationship Between Cholesterol and Heart Disease Mortality

Lower cholesterol levels are easily attainable by limiting or cutting out red meat, eggs, poultry, and all dairy products, junk foods, and fried foods from your diet. People who are genetically predisposed to high cholesterol levels can still easily keep them under 200 mg/dL with just a few changes to their diet and lifestyle. Make sure that no more than 20 percent of your daily calories come from fat; less than 15 percent is even better. Also, watch your intake of vegetable oils, as excessive consumption is harmful to cardiovascular health. Remember to have regular blood serum tests to keep your levels in check.

TRIGLYCERIDES

Another type of lipid found in the blood, *triglycerides* are stored in the body's fat cells and used for energy. In terms of cardiovascular health, the triglyceride count is the second most meaningful blood lipid value after cholesterol. (For diabetes and other blood sugar issues, your triglycerides level is the most important blood lipid value.) High triglyceride levels can increase your chances of developing *metabolic syndrome,* a group of disorders that typically occur together and raise the risk of heart disease, as well as type 2 diabetes and stroke.

Triglyceride levels are raised by consuming foods high in sugar. Sweets of all kinds, including sources of natural sugar like honey and maple syrup, will also raise your triglycerides, even if you are following an otherwise low-fat diet. Although vegans and vegetarians may have lower cholesterol than meat eaters, they are at equal risk for elevated triglycerides due to their intake of various sugars. It's not sufficient to stay away from only white processed sugar; you also must avoid natural sugars found in agave, dried fruit, and fruit juices, among other sources.

Avoiding foods containing hydrogenated oils, also called trans fats or partially hydrogenated oils, is important for controlling triglycerides as well. Over the past few decades, there have been numerous studies from around the world confirming the harmful effects of these substances. Hydrogenated oils are made by extracting cheap oils, such as cottonseed oil, and, under extreme pressure and heat, forcing hydrogen gas into them with a platinum catalyst. Margarine and shortening are two major sources of hydrogenated oils. Contrary to popular belief, margarine is not "better" than butter; in fact, it is worse. You can buy non-hydrogenated non-dairy spreads made of coconut and palm oils temporarily as you make the transition to not using butter or margarine at all, which is ideal. Also be aware that vegetable oils can be just as harmful as hydrogenated oils. Read the nutrition labels on every packaged food you buy to make sure the word "hydrogenated" is not listed. Keep in mind that eating in fast food restaurants is risky, since the types of oils and fats used in their foods are not mentioned on the menu, for obvious reasons. When you eat at a restaurant, it's practically guaranteed that you will be consuming trans fats.

Although any value less than 150 mg/dL is considered normal by most doctors, triglyceride levels should actually be kept under 100 mg/dL. Regular blood testing will help you monitor your level.

HOMOCYSTEINE

Homocysteine (Hcy) is an amino acid used by the body to maintain tissues and make proteins. Homocysteine is a key diagnostic factor when it comes to evaluating cardiovascular health, as it's strongly correlated with all forms of coronary heart disease (CHD). Therefore, it's important that you have your level tested regularly. Blood homocysteine levels tend to increase as you age, and men generally have higher levels than women. Smoking, drinking coffee, high cholesterol, and hypertension (high blood pressure), as well as mental disorders like depression and dementia, are all associated with raised homocysteine. People with diabetes and insulin resistance also have high levels of homocysteine.

Like cholesterol and triglycerides, homocysteine levels are higher among populations of Western countries due to diet and lifestyle factors. Studies have shown that the Westernized diet plays a decisive role in raising levels. One study found that the average level among Mexicans living in rural areas of their native Mexico was 9 mmol/L, while those living in urban areas with access to "Western" foods high in fat and sugar had an average level of 12 mmol/L. A level over 15 mmol/L is considered to be pathological (hyperhomocystemia), as it doubles the risk and incidence of coronary heart disease.

It's possible to lower homocysteine with a triple supplement containing vitamin B_6 (2 mg), B_{12} (1 mg in the form of methylcobalamin), and folic acid (800 mcg). However, this effect is superficial, since the supplement has not been shown to actually reduce CHD occurrence. This was demonstrated in a study done at McMaster University in Canada, where 5,522 people were given the triple supplement for five years. Although homocysteine levels decreased considerably, there was no reduction in the incidence of coronary heart disease. A more effective method is to take 1,000 mg (two doses of 500 mg) of trimethylglycine (TMG) daily, follow a whole grain-based diet, and adopt healthy lifestyle practices. Maintain a level on the lower end of the normal range, which is 5 to 15 mmol/L. A level below 10 mmol/L is ideal.

C-REACTIVE PROTEIN

C-reactive protein (CRP) is a protein in the blood that becomes elevated when inflammation is present in the body. Causes of inflammation range from minor infections and burns to serious medical conditions such as obesity, diabetes, cancer, and heart problems. In general, the hs-CRP (high sensitivity) test is an accurate predictor of coronary heart disease, as well as diabetes and arthritis. Other factors associated with high CRP levels include high uric acid (see below), hypertension, insulin resistance, smoking, obesity, lack of exercise, use of oral contraceptives, and high homocysteine, total cholesterol, and triglycerides. Those living in rural areas of Asian countries tend to have very low CRP levels due to their low-fat diets and physical labor. Among the US population, African Americans generally have the highest CRP levels.

As always, the best way to lower your CRP level is with diet and lifestyle modifications. This means following a low-sugar, low-fat diet of natural foods that reduces inflammation in your body. Exercising, losing weight, reducing alcohol intake, quitting smoking, and avoiding birth control pills and prescription drugs will also help lower CRP. Taking a complete mineral supplement, multivitamin, and the other nutritional supplements listed in Chapter 16 (see page 117) is recommended as well. It is very important that you have an hs-CRP test. The average range is 1.0 to 3.0 mg/L, but an optimal level is 1.0 or under.

URIC ACID

A common misconception about *uric acid*, a chemical created during digestion, is that eating foods high in purines will raise levels. However, it is actually the consumption of animal proteins and fats that is responsible for elevating uric acid. This includes red meats, poultry, eggs, and milk, as well as dairy products, which do not contain purines. The fact that vegetarians, vegans, and people who follow macrobiotic diets all have low uric acid levels is proof that animal products are the real culprit. Asians—especially those in China, Japan, Thailand, and Vietnam—have the lowest levels of any population in the world and eat the least amount of animal products. Meanwhile, the US population has the highest uric acid levels overall due to a diet high in red meat, dairy, and sugar, which can also raise UA.

High uric acid is correlated with hypertension, diabetes, insulin resistance, metabolic syndrome, low HDL, high LDL, raised triglycerides, obesity, high blood sugar and insulin, atherosclerosis (hardening and narrowing of arteries), and heart disease in general. A study from the Spokane Heart

Institute shows that people with UA levels over 5.2 mg/dL have more than three times the risk of dying from cardiovascular disease. The most stunning study of all is from the Radiation Effects Foundation in Japan (*Journal of Rheumatology*, v. 32, 2005), which observed 10,615 people over twenty-five years. It found that high uric acid levels are correlated with all-cause mortality, meaning that people with high UA are more likely to die from every known cause.

Make sure to have your uric acid tested regularly. An optimal level for women is any number below 4.0 mg/dL, and for men, 5.0 mg/dL. The ranges generally accepted as "normal" for uric acid are not ideal.

SUPPLEMENTS FOR HEART HEALTH

Dietary modification is necessary for maintaining ideal levels of cholesterol, triglycerides, homocysteine, CRP, and uric acid. If you are willing to make better food choices and exercise regularly, the results can be truly astounding. Prescription drugs are not necessary; in fact, taking them can be a very unwise and ineffective approach to dealing with high cholesterol and raised levels of the other blood values mentioned in this chapter. The drugs that are commonly prescribed are not effective, very expensive, and have severe side effects. They also do not lengthen your lifespan and actually worsen your health. It is very easy to lower your cholesterol and triglyceride levels naturally without dangerous toxic drugs. Four cornerstone nutritional supplements, when used along with diet and exercise, can be hugely beneficial for lowering levels of cholesterol and triglycerides, reducing your overall risk of heart disease, and boosting your general health. These four supplements—beta glucan, beta-sitosterol, flaxseed oil, and soy isoflavones—are discussed below.

Beta Glucan

This substance—which is found in foods such as oats, cereal grains, baker's (brewer's) yeast, and mushrooms—is the most powerful immune enhancer known to science, as it activates the cells that trigger the body's immune response. Research on beta glucan dates back three decades, so its health benefits are well documented. Studies have shown that the substance can significantly improve cholesterol and triglyceride levels, which does wonders for your heart, and its potent anti-cancer properties are currently being studied. Technological advancements in the last few years have made it possible to easily extract beta glucan from various sources, so it is readily available to the public and inexpensive. You can use either yeast or oat beta glucan, as both are equally effective. However, eating barley or oatmeal several times a week will allow you to get all the benefits of beta glucan, so taking supplements is not necessary.

Recommended Dosage: 200 to 400 mg per day.

Beta-Sitosterol

Beta-sitosterol is a type of plant sterol found in practically every vegetable, but most Americans do not get enough of it from their regular dietary intake. It is estimated that the average American adult consumes about 300 mg of beta-sitosterol daily, while vegetarians eat twice this amount. This substance, which has been known about for over forty years, has powerful and beneficial effects on blood lipids that have been verified by published international studies. Beta-sitosterol is contained in mixed plant sterol supplements, which are the single most important heart-healthy natural supplements you can take.

Recommended Dosage: 300 mg to 600 mg per day.

Flaxseed Oil

Flaxseed oil, which is extracted from the seeds of the flax plant, is the single best source of omega-3 fatty acids. The standard Western diet includes far too many omega-6 fatty acids (*linoleic acids*) due to the fact that so many foods are cooked in and prepared with vegetable oils—a chief source of omega-6. However, most people do not get enough omega-3s (*linolenic acids*). The amount of research on the benefits of omega-3s for heart health and blood lipid levels is overwhelming, yet deficiency is an epidemic. There are many studies confirming the varied health benefits of flaxseed oil, including improved blood lipid levels and cardiovascular health. Supplements are available in bulk or in capsule form. Buy only refrigerated flaxseed oil, as unrefrigerated flaxseed oil oxidizes easily, and keep it refrigerated.

Recommended Dosage: 1,000 to 2,000 mg (one to two capsules) per day, or $1/2$-tsp of bulk flaxseed oil.

Soy Isoflavones

Soy isoflavones are compounds derived from soybeans and other soy products. However, not all forms of soy are created equal. Tofu is the white bread of soybeans, as it is highly refined and lacking in nutrients, and soy sauce is merely a condiment. Traditional Asian dishes contain healthy sources of soy, such as miso, seitan, tempeh, and soy flour, but Westerners rarely consume these foods. The Japanese (particularly Okinawans) eat more soy than any other population in the world and enjoy the longest lifespan, which reflects the value of soy isoflavones. There is an overwhelming amount of published studies on the positive effects of soy supplementation for a variety of diseases and conditions, including heart disease. Yet, the amount you need to see any benefits is more than you will be able to get just by eating soy-containing foods. You would have to drink 1 cup of soy milk per day, and this will add a whopping 3,600 calories to your daily intake per month, as most brands contain an average of 120 calories per serving. This is why supplementation is a better way to meet your body's needs for soy isoflavones. Use a supplement that contains mixed isoflavones, particularly genestein and daidzein.

Recommended Dosage: 40 mg per day.

If you are over forty years of age, there are other supplements you should be taking in addition to the four supplements discussed here. Chapters 16 and 17 (see pages 117 and 131) contain more information about these supplements, which include acetyl-L-carnitine (ALC), acidophilus (a probiotic), beta carotene, coenzyme Q_{10} (CoQ_{10}), diindolylmethane (DIM), fructooligosaccharides (FOS), glucosamine, L-glutamine, lipoic acid, N-acetylcysteine (NAC), phosphatidylserine (PS), quercetin, vitamins D and E, and a number of essential minerals. If you are under forty years old, you need only take acidophilus, beta glucan, flaxseed oil, FOS, L-glutamine, vitamins D and E, a multivitamin, and a complete mineral supplement.

HORMONE BALANCE AND YOUR HEART

In addition to diet and supplements, hormone balance plays an important role in cardiovascular health and the circulatory system. One of the primary functions of cholesterol is producing hormones, including DHEA, pregnenolone, testosterone, progesterone, androstenedione, estradiol, estrone, and estriol. Deficient or excessive hormone levels interfere with cholesterol metabolism. Doctors usually do not take into account the fact that your basic hormones strongly affect cholesterol and triglyceride levels, so hormone tests are not typically administered to patients with high lipid levels.

In 2002, the Mississippi Regional Cancer Center published a study entitled, "Hypercholesterolemia Treatment: A New Hypothesis" (*Medical Hypotheses*, v. 59, 2002). A group of progressive doctors treated patients with high cholesterol and triglycerides by balancing their basic hormones using bioidentical DHEA, testosterone, T3, T4, pregnenolone, progesterone, estradiol, estrone, estriol, and cortisol. Results of the study showed that balancing the entire endocrine system has a significant positive effect on blood lipids and, therefore, cardiovascular health.

If you are over forty years of age, you definitely need to test and balance your levels of estrogen (all three), testosterone, DHEA, progesterone, pregnenolone, and melatonin, as well as your thyroid hormones T3 and T4. However, growth hormone (GH) therapy has shown little benefit for heart and artery health, and is very overrated. People over fifty years of age can take GH injections if they can afford it, but it's more important to focus on balancing your other hormones.

CONCLUSION

Although heart disease is currently the number one cause of death among women in the United States, steps can be taken to reverse this trend. Furthermore, preventing and treating heart disease can and should be done naturally. Diet, supplements, and proper hormone balance will allow you to keep your blood lipid levels within normal ranges and maintain good cardiovascular health. Also remember that that you need exercise in order to keep your heart strong and your arteries clear, as well as to maintain a healthy weight and general wellness. Even walking for thirty minutes a day will do the job. Decades ago, the nutritionist Nathan Pritikin worked miracles with heart patients by keeping them on a low-fat, high-fiber, whole grain-based diet and having them walk five miles per day. Ideally, though, you should try to do a combination of aerobic and resistance exercise. Together, these four elements—diet, supplements, hormone balance, and exercise—create a total lifestyle program for keeping your heart and arteries in the best of health, and in a completely natural way.

12. Diabetes

Diabetes is the fastest growing disease in the world. Currently, one in every ten people has diabetes in the United States, and the number is increasing. One in three American children will grow up diabetic. It is also on the rise in Europe, Australia, India, Japan, and China, and there are millions who live with the disease unknowingly. According to the most recent statistics, more than 10 percent of American women over the age of twenty have diabetes, and the rate of *gestational diabetes*—diabetes induced by pregnancy—is increasing. Furthermore, *insulin resistance,* a precursor to diabetes, is also an epidemic and affects more men, women, and children each year. Diabetes and insulin resistance can lead to a number of different medical conditions, including heart disease, stroke, high blood pressure, and a host of other problems. This is why it's so crucial to reverse the disease or, better yet, stop it before it happens—which you *can* do. After reading this chapter, you will understand why the rate of diabetes is increasing at such a rapid rate, putting you in a much better position to prevent it from affecting you and diminishing your health.

ABOUT DIABETES

Diabetes is a group of diseases that affect how the body uses *blood glucose,* or blood sugar, which is a major source of energy for your cells. In general, diabetes is characterized by an excess of glucose in the blood, leading to health problems. *Type 1 diabetes*, formerly known as *juvenile diabetes* or *insulin-dependent diabetes*, is a chronic condition in which the pancreas is unable to produce *insulin,* the hormone that is needed to allow glucose to enter the cells and produce energy. Type 1 accounts for only about 5 to 10 percent of diabetes cases, and is more common in Caucasians and young people, appearing most often during adolescence. It is typically caused by genetic, autoimmune, or environmental factors, and there is currently no way to cure it. However, it can be effectively managed with insulin injections, and quality of life can be dramatically improved by following the lifestyle guidelines in this chapter (see page 94).

Type 2 diabetes is the type most people are referring to when talking about diabetes, accounting for 90 to 95 percent of diabetes cases among adults. It is more common in African Americans, Latinos, Native Americans, and Asian Americans, as well as older people. It is also strongly associated with poor diet, lack of physical activity, family history, and obesity. Once known as *adult-onset diabetes,* or *non-insulin-dependent diabetes,* type 2 occurs when the cells do not respond to insulin properly (insulin resistance). As the body starts to require more and more insulin to maintain normal blood sugar levels, the pancreas slowly loses its ability to produce insulin. Type 2 diabetes often leads to serious health problems that can be life-threatening, like heart disease. However, the condition is highly preventable and can be effectively treated, usually within a year or less.

Gestational diabetes, the third type, is a form of glucose intolerance that occurs during pregnancy. It affects women who do not have a history of diabetes, and blood sugar regulation generally returns to normal after giving birth. However, the risk of developing type 2 diabetes later in life increases after being diagnosed with gestational diabetes, which causes pregnancy complications if left untreated.

In general, diabetes affects many parts of the body, and can lead to blindness, kidney damage, periodontal disease, nervous system damage, limb amputations, heart disease, and stroke. It also produces symptoms like chronic fatigue, physical weakness, increased thirst and urination, and slow-healing wounds. Type 2 diabetes in particular is associated with *metabolic syndrome,* as well as *prediabetes,* which are quickly becoming epidemics in the United States.

METABOLIC SYNDROME AND PREDIABETES

Prediabetes is a condition characterized by blood sugar levels that are higher than normal, but not high enough to be considered full diabetes. According to studies, people who are prediabetic will develop type 2 diabetes within a decade unless they lose weight. Prediabetes does not have any symptoms, so the only way to know if you have it is by getting a blood test (see page 93). However, it may occur in conjunction with disorders that collectively make up the condition known as *metabolic syndrome,* formerly called Syndrome X, which increases the risk of type 2 diabetes. In addition to high blood glucose levels, metabolic syndrome is characterized by:

- Dyslipidemia, or abnormal levels of cholesterol and triglycerides in the blood, which increases the risk of heart and blood vessel damage

- Hypertension (high blood pressure)

- Insulin resistance

- Obesity or excess weight, particularly around the waist

Age and race are also factors in metabolic syndrome. The risk of the condition increases as you get older, and there is a greater risk among Asians and Hispanics. The Centers for Disease Control and Prevention (CDC) recently studied 8,814 normal men and women. They found that 22 percent of them exhibited at least three of the conditions that make up metabolic syndrome. Moreover, 44 percent of people over the age of sixty had at least three of the conditions. This means that almost *half* of Americans over sixty are prediabetic, and most do not realize it.

DIAGNOSING DIABETES

An ounce of prevention is worth ten pounds of cure. In order to prevent the disease, you must get certain basic diagnostic tests, which are also beneficial for your overall health. In addition to a standard blood analysis—which should include glucose, total cholesterol, HDL cholesterol, LDL cholesterol, triglycerides, uric acid, C-reactive protein (CRP), homocysteine, and creatinine—you should have at least one of these blood sugar tests:

- **Fasting Blood Sugar (FBS).** This is the most common blood sugar test and requires fasting—abstaining from eating and all beverages except water—for at least eight hours beforehand. Although most doctors consider values less than 100 mg/dL to be "normal," levels really should be kept under 85 mg/dL (4.7 mmol/L). International research has shown that people with blood sugar levels under 85 mg/dL are healthier and live longer than those with levels over 85 mg/dL. Accurate and inexpensive at-home blood sugar meters are available in pharmacies and drugstores. Good brands include TRUEbalance and TRUEtest, which can be purchased for as little as ten dollars.

- **Glucose Tolerance Test (GTT).** Also known as the oral glucose tolerance test, the GTT measures your body's response to glucose. Once your fast-

ing blood sugar level is determined, you are asked to drink 50 g of a glucose solution. After waiting one hour, your blood sugar is measured
again to record the change in your level. This test also indicates how well
your muscles respond to insulin. The GTT is underutilized and used
mostly to diagnose gestational diabetes, but it is safe, non-invasive, and
inexpensive. Always measure your level using a number that is twenty
points under the accepted medical standard. In other words, if the generally accepted "normal" level is 140 mg/dL, you want to keep your
level at 120 mg/dL or under.

- **HbA1c (Glycated Hemoglobin) Test.** This optional test measures long-
  term *glycation*, or the accumulation of sugar molecules in your blood's
  hemoglobin over a six-month period. An ideal number for this is 4.7 percent (the equivalent of a fasting blood sugar level of 85 mg/dL) or under,
  not 5.6 percent (100 mg/dL), which is the accepted medical standard.
  This is a good test, but unnecessary if you have a GTT. It can be purchased inexpensively at chain drugstores.

The best blood sugar test is the glucose tolerance test. In addition to this
test and a standard blood analysis, you should also measure your blood
pressure, which should be kept at 120/80 or less. You may also want to
have the liver assays SGOT/AST and SGPT/ALT (aspartate aminotransferase and alanine aminotransferase) measured. An albumin urine test to
check your kidney function is also a good idea, since kidney dysfunction is
one of the most common severe side effects of diabetes.

PREVENTING AND TREATING DIABETES NATURALLY

Scientists are in agreement that insulin and blood sugar dysfunction is due
largely to *oxidative stress,* a condition in which *free radicals*—highly reactive
molecules that cause damage to cells—run rampant throughout the body
and must be counteracted by *antioxidants,* protective substances that work
to prevent oxidation. This uses up the body's supply of antioxidants, a
group that includes glutathione, superoxide dismutase (SOD), beta carotene, vitamins C and E, CoQ_{10}, melatonin, and lipoic acid, among others.
Oxidative stress is strongly associated with poor diet and lifestyle, which is
why better food choices and general healthy living is needed to lower it
and, in turn, normalize your blood sugar.

The most important thing to do is to modify your diet. Americans eat
more than double the amount of calories they need; men need only about
1,800 calories per day, and women require approximately 1,200 calories. You

can simultaneously cut your caloric intake and improve your blood glucose levels if you stop eating all forms of sugar, including sweeteners—even ones that manufacturers claim to be "natural." All simple sugars are essentially the same, whether it's maltose, fructose, sucrose, white sugar, brown sugar, or raw sugar, or from fruit juice, dried fruit, agave, molasses, honey, maple syrup, corn syrup, or amazake. You must also cut out sugar substitutes, including aspartame, lo han, stevia, and sucralose. Until your blood sugar is normal, do not eat any sweets. This may sound extreme, but it is necessary, as your body is unable to digest and metabolize simple sugars properly when you have blood glucose problems. This applies even to fruits, which are devoid of meaningful amounts of just about every known nutrient.

You must also remove all excess fat, especially saturated fat, from your diet. As mentioned already, most Americans get a whopping 42 percent of their daily calories from saturated fats, which raises cholesterol and triglycerides. Diabetics almost always have abnormal blood lipid levels. Stop eating all red meat, poultry, eggs, and dairy products, even ones that are low-fat or nonfat. Remember that dairy products contain indigestible lactose and the cancer-promoting substance casein. Your diet should be mostly from plants with some seafood (about 10 percent), as long as you are not allergic to it. A pure vegetarian diet is also a good option. Use very little vegetable oil, which is a source of fat. Ideally, no more than 10 percent of your daily calories should come from fats (from vegetable sources only), but 15 percent is acceptable.

In addition to vegetables, your diet should be based on whole grains and beans. Replace white rice, white bread, white pasta, and white flour with grains like brown rice, whole wheat, barley, spelt, quinoa, oats, rye, millet, and buckwheat. Beans and yellow and green vegetables (except nightshades) are also good for you. All of these foods digest and metabolize very slowly, which means that they fill you up and prevent you from consuming empty calories. Over time, these foods also help normalize blood sugar levels. In 2002, researchers at the University of Minnesota conducted a study of 160,000 people and found that a diet based largely on whole grains significantly reduced the incidence of diabetes. A study from the National Public Health Institute of Finland in 2003, which analyzed almost 5,000 people, produced the same findings, as did Harvard University and the USDA. Furthermore, in 2001, scientists at South Korea's Yonsei University found that people could lower their blood sugar by an amazing 24 percent in just sixteen weeks by eating whole grains. The famous Framingham Heart Study also identified a link between eating whole grains and the prevention and treatment of diabetes.

The central role that diet plays in preventing diabetes and blood sugar problems is perhaps best shown by the Pima Indians, who live in both Mexico and Arizona. The Pimas in Mexico are slim, generally very healthy, and have low rates of heart disease and diabetes. They eat a traditional diet of corn, beans, vegetables, and other natural foods, and consume very little meat, sugar, and refined foods. The Pimas in Arizona, on the other hand, are a different case. They have high rates of overweight and obesity, high cholesterol levels, heart disease, and diabetes. Not surprisingly, they eat a typical American diet of red meat, sweets, and processed foods. This is real-world proof that a healthy diet based on natural foods can prevent diabetes and a host of other health problems.

Lifestyle is also vital. Since nicotine, alcohol, and caffeine can add to oxidative stress and, therefore, high blood sugar, you should end bad habits like smoking, drinking alcohol, and consuming coffee. Exercise is another important lifestyle component, and it is absolutely necessary for treating, preventing, and managing blood sugar conditions. If you want to cure diabetes, you must exercise, even if it's just by walking for thirty minutes a day. You can do aerobic or resistance exercise, but a combination of both is ideal. The more you exercise, the more quickly you will improve your condition, as well as achieve and maintain good health. Studies from Harvard University, University of Perugia, University of Barcelona, University of Vienna, Syracuse University, Maastricht University, University of Maryland, and other world-renowned institutions have all confirmed the link between regular exercise and the management and prevention of diabetes, along with insulin resistance and other blood sugar problems. Plus, physical activity promotes weight loss, and most people with type 2 diabetes are overweight or obese, which contributes to high blood sugar and other conditions like heart disease. Simply put, if you are diabetic (or prediabetic) and overweight, you must lose excess pounds in order to normalize your blood sugar and insulin. There is no way around it.

Natural supplements and hormones also contribute to overall health. Doctors usually prescribe allopathic drug treatments that address the symptoms of the condition rather than the cause. These synthetic toxins just make the condition worse, and they have many serious side effects, such as severe liver and kidney damage and lactic acid buildup. Instead of taking potentially harmful medications, take the nutritional supplements discussed in Chapter 16 (see page 117). Men and women over the age of forty should take all twenty supplements. Supplementing with antioxidants like beta carotene, lipoic acid, vitamins C and E, and CoQ_{10} is important for neutralizing the free radicals that cause oxidative stress. Bioidentical hormone supplements may be necessary as well, since hormone imbalances are common in diabetics and people with blood sugar conditions. After all, insulin is a basic hormone that works synergistically with other vital hormones, like DHEA, testosterone, pregnenolone, estriol, and thyroid hormones T3 and T4. Yet, despite the medical studies verifying the link, hormone imbalance is rarely considered as a factor in diabetes. Make sure you ask to have your levels tested.

Although fasting (abstaining from all foods and drinks except water) for one day per week is recommended for most people, diabetics are unable to fast for more than a few hours without becoming ill. However, by following these lifestyle guidelines, your condition will improve, allowing you to fast for longer and longer periods of time without experiencing any adverse side effects or discomfort. When you are off all diabetes medications, you can fast for a full twenty-four hours—and gradually even longer—without any problems.

Type 2 diabetes can be cured within a year or less with the right diet, supplements, regular exercise, and hormone balance. Once you begin following the guidelines discussed above, you will see clear improvements in your blood sugar levels and overall health every month. Some people have even been able to cure themselves in less than six months. However, type 1 diabetes, for which there is currently no cure, cannot be managed through diet and lifestyle alone. This is because type 1 diabetes is caused by an impaired or atrophied pancreas, forcing those who have the condition to take insulin for the rest of their lives. Beta cell and pancreas transplants simply do not work. These people can, however, make dramatic improvements in health and longevity, as well as reduce their insulin needs, by making better dietary and lifestyle choices.

CONCLUSION

Of the millions of people who have been diagnosed with diabetes in the United States, more than half are women. And with the rising rates of heart disease and obesity, this number will certainly increase. Although diabetes is a burden on all people who have it, the disease presents unique problems for women because of its effect on the menstrual cycle and pregnancy. Moreover, only women, not men, can be affected by gestational diabetes, which raises the risk of developing type 2 diabetes later in life. Therefore, it is especially important for women to control their blood sugar naturally by eating a balanced diet and practicing healthy living. Simply by choosing the right foods and avoiding the wrong ones, exercising, taking supplements, and keeping your hormones in balance, you can ward off this epidemic and spare yourself numerous health problems.

13. Obesity

I t's no secret that the United States is the fattest nation in the world. We've come a long way from 1970s TV shows, in which everyone appears healthy and slim. Today, the majority of the population is medically defined as overweight, more than 30 percent of Americans are clinically obese, and the number of overweight teenagers and young children continues to increase. As a result, dieting has become a huge industry, with many popular fad diets targeted specifically at women. Yet, obesity rates continue to climb, due to factors such as poor food choices and eating habits, sedentary lifestyle, and a misguided belief in short-term fad diets. Obesity has become a national trend and medical crisis, as numerous health risks are associated with excess weight. This chapter takes a closer look at our growing weight problem and gives you the information you need to prevent obesity, lose weight, and keep off unhealthy pounds.

OBESITY IN THE UNITED STATES

Obesity is clinically defined as an excess of body fat, and is measured by the body mass index (BMI), which is a calculation based on an individual's height and weight. Obesity is linked to practically every disease on the rise today, including cancer, type 2 diabetes, insulin resistance, liver disease, kidney disease, high blood pressure, heart disease, inflammation, sleep apnea, depression, and various psychological problems. In women, obesity can lead to menstrual irregularities and pregnancy complications. It is also associated with high blood lipid levels, elevated blood sugar and insulin, high homocysteine, high CRP, high uric acid, increased oxidative stress, lowered immunity, and early death. Recent statistics show that over two-thirds of American adults are obese or overweight—including 64 percent of women—and over one-third are considered medically obese. This condition has already started to affect children, who are developing more chronic health problems at a younger age.

There are several factors that contribute to obesity, including high calorie intake, poor diet, and lack of exercise. To a lesser extent, genetics, illness, and hormonal imbalance play a role; these factors can account for *some*, but not all, excess pounds. An underactive thyroid can cause weight gain, so you should have your free T3 and T4 levels checked if you are having difficulty losing weight. Overweight and obese women have been shown to have high levels of estrone and estradiol, but are universally low in estriol. As explained in Chapter 3, you can test your level of estriol with an at-home saliva testing kit, since doctors rarely measure it. The only way to lower estrone and estradiol is with a low-fat and high-fiber diet based on whole grains, exercise, and other lifestyle changes, such as avoiding alcohol. Another hormone that is often influential in weight gain is insulin, so you should have a GTT (see page 93) to determine your insulin metabolism. (See page 94 to learn how to normalize your blood sugar and insulin levels naturally.) Be sure to regularly measure your hormones so that you can keep them balanced and allow them to work together synergistically.

Still, the main reason why Westerners, particularly Americans, are becoming increasingly overweight is the consumption of excessive amounts of saturated fat, sugar, and nutrition-less processed foods. The combination of an unhealthy diet and poor eating habits has created a nation in which weight loss is needed not only to boost physical fitness and confidence, but to prevent serious and potentially life-threatening diseases.

A NATURAL DIET VERSUS "DIETING"

Following a natural diet is completely different from "dieting." Contrary to popular belief, you do not have to go hungry in order to lose weight. Not only is this unhealthy and unnecessary, but it also goes against our human instincts. Do you know a single person who can abstain from food for several hours at a time and not feel any desire to eat? Eating is essential for staying alive and engrained in us. The key to weight loss is not being hungry all the time, but rather making better food choices.

It's important to eat only when you are actually hungry. Real hunger can be satisfied with something small and simple, such as a piece of whole-grain bread with apple butter or a piece of fruit that is low in sugar. If you are craving chocolate cake instead of whole natural foods, you are looking for emotional, not physical, satisfaction. You should follow a diet of whole grains, beans, vegetables (preferably green and yellow), healthy soups and salads, and moderate amounts of fruit and seafood. Meat, poultry, eggs, dairy, processed foods, and foods containing sugar should be eliminated. It's also a good idea to get in the habit of eating a bowl of hot hearty soup before lunch and dinner. Soup tends to be low in fat and calories, and it fills you up so that you consume less food during the meal, in turn reducing your calorie intake. Hot soup before a meal is a tradition in Asian cultures— yet another reason why they are some of the slimmest, healthiest people in the world. You can find plenty of recipes for nutritious, tasty soups in a cookbook. When you make better food choices and practice healthy eating habits, you will be consuming fewer calories every day from nutrient-rich sources. You will reap more health benefits, facilitate weight loss, and never feel deprived. In fact, you will be able to eat just as much—if not more— food than you were previously.

Dr. Terry Shintani led a study at the University of Hawaii (*American Journal of Clinical Nutrition* v. 53, 1991) in which native Hawaiians in very poor health were put on a traditional diet high in complex carbohydrates and low in fat, with moderate amounts of protein. They ate everything they wanted, including taro, breadfruit, yams, green vegetables, local fruit, seafood, and even some chicken. (Hawaiians traditionally eat root vegetables rather than grains.) In just three weeks, the patients lost an average of 17 pounds each, and dramatically lowered their blood pressure, cholesterol, and blood sugar. These results, which were achieved through dietary changes alone (not supplements or exercise), is real-world proof that you can eat what you want and maintain a healthy weight as long as you make smart food choices. Food does not make you fat; fat makes you fat.

The positive correlation between a low-fat diet and weight loss was also demonstrated in a human clinical study at Cornell University (*American Journal of Clinical Nutrition*, v. 46, 1987). All the people who participated in the study were given the same foods, but they varied the amount of fat calories. For example, every person was given bran muffins, but some were loaded with fattening ingredients like butter and eggs, while others were not. They were allowed to eat as much as they wanted without restriction. The researchers found that those who ate the low-fat versions of foods consumed 2,087 calories a day, while the people who were given the foods high in fat ate 2,714 calories. Based on the results of this two-week study, the researchers calculated that the healthy group could expect to lose 23 pounds in a year, while the unhealthy group would *gain* about 18 pounds in a year. Once again, it is fat—not food in general—that causes weight gain.

A study from the University of Alabama (*American Journal of Clinical Nutrition*, v. 37, 1983) assessed the total caloric intake of people who were given unrestricted access to foods varying in fat content. The people were not weighed, as the doctors wanted to only determine calorie consumption. The study found that the people who ate low-fat foods took in an average of 1,570 calories per day, even though they could eat as much as they wanted. Those who ate high-fat foods, however, consumed nearly double that amount, averaging 3,000 calories per day. This is the power of better food choices.

A real-life example is the typical diet of many populations in rural parts of Asia. Although they subsist mainly on vegetables and grains, such as rice, wheat, and barley, these people surprisingly tend to have a high calorie consumption. However, because their calories are coming from natural sources rather than animal products, dairy, and refined foods, obesity is uncommon, as are most forms of cancer, diabetes, heart disease, and other chronic conditions. Of course, this limited diet is forced upon them due to their location and lifestyle, but they are nevertheless healthier than Americans, who are generally wealthier and more privileged. Interestingly, though, there is a higher rate of disease among people who live in the urban areas of countries like China, Indonesia, Japan, and Thailand, since many of them have adopted the Western diet. As they consume more beef, pork, chicken, milk, cheese, butter, eggs, and other high-calorie and high-fat foods, their health deteriorates at a proportional rate, and the incidence of disease has become similar to that of Western countries.

These studies clearly demonstrate that the standard high-fat Western diet is the main culprit when it comes to overweight and obesity. Simply by eliminating saturated fats, sugars, and refined foods, and replacing them with more vegetables and whole grains, you will significantly lower your calorie consumption and increase your intake of valuable nutrients. This will also allow you to eat more without going over your daily calorie needs, as well as to stay satisfied.

EXERCISE

Exercise is essential for facilitating and maintaining weight loss. There is no way around it. Even if you eat the right foods, maintain hormone balance, and take a variety of beneficial supplements, you still need to exercise in order to keep weight off, improve your physical fitness, and promote overall wellness. In addition to combating disease, exercise also boosts your energy level and mood.

A combination of both *aerobic exercise* and *resistance exercise* is ideal. Aerobic exercise is any moderate to intense activity that is done for an extended period of time, raises your heart rate and oxygen needs, and involves multiple muscle groups. In addition to strengthening your cardiovascular system, aerobic exercise improves immunity, reduces fatigue, and lowers certain health risks, such as obesity, heart disease, high blood pressure, stroke, type 2 diabetes, and some cancers. One of the best, easiest, and most enjoyable forms of aerobic exercise is walking, which is recommended for people with health conditions like diabetes, as well as for individuals who are just beginning an exercise regimen. A thirty-minute walk per day is all you need to reap health benefits. Gradually, you can build the length and intensity of each session, or you can engage in higher-intensity activities such as jogging, swimming, bicycling, dancing, or using an elliptical or rowing machine. You should always practice caution when starting a new activity or beginning to work out at a higher level of intensity.

Resistance exercise, which is also called strength training, is done to increase the strength and mass of your bones and muscle. This helps to prevent conditions like osteoporosis, increase HDL ("good" cholesterol) levels, and reduce body fat. Since muscle burns more calories than fat, resistance exercise also improves your metabolism, making it particularly beneficial for losing and managing your weight. A resistance workout can be done with weight machines, free weights, or even your own body weight with calisthenics like sit-ups, push-ups, and chin-ups. As with aerobic exercise, you can steadily increase the length and intensity of your workout over time as long as you practice caution.

Although exercise is only part of a weight-loss plan, it is absolutely necessary if you want to keep off the weight you lose. Even with the right diet, weight loss will be temporary unless you are physically active. Moreover, you need to exercise in order to maintain a good level of fitness, which contributes to your general health and well-being.

CONCLUSION

The only way to achieve and maintain a healthy weight is through diet and lifestyle change. Popular diet books and fad diets—such as those based on the glycemic index—simply do not work. If they did, obesity wouldn't be such a huge problem in the United States and other Western countries. There are also no magic supplements to help you lose weight, despite the billions of dollars worth of supposed diet aids that are sold every year. Furthermore, amphetamine-based drugs prescribed for weight loss are effective only in the short-term, and are accompanied by a number of psychological, emotional, and physical side effects. It is up to you to use the information and advice in this book, as well as the recommended books listed on page 147, to make lasting lifestyle changes that will enable you to shed excess pounds and keep them off. Eating mindfully, choosing whole natural foods, and exercising are three basic ingredients not only for weight loss, but also for general wellness. You will never be hungry when you eat whole natural foods. Remember, weight loss does not require "willpower," but rather an understanding of your body and how to achieve total health.

14. Natural Diet

As emphasized throughout this book, nearly every major illness and medical condition from osteoporosis to breast cancer is linked in some way to diet. Simply put, diet is everything. Nothing is more important to your health than what you eat every day. The saying is true: you *are* what you eat. And Americans—women as well as men—eat more than double the amount of calories and animal protein they need, and more than six times the amount of fat. Americans also consume an average of 160 pounds of sugar annually, and barely get half of the necessary fiber, vitamins, minerals, and other vital nutrients. In other words, almost everyone in the United States unknowingly suffers from chronic nutritional deficiency, which explains the prevalence of conditions like obesity, heart disease, type 2 diabetes, and cancer. There are far lower rates of these diseases in countries like Japan, where the typical diet is based primarily on vegetables, soy foods, and fish. This just goes to show that you can prevent disease and preserve your overall wellness by adopting a healthy diet of natural foods. This chapter takes a look at several food groups, highlighting commonly consumed foods that promote disease while guiding you in choosing the right foods to support vitality and longevity.

MEAT, POULTRY, AND EGGS

Americans get about 42 percent of their daily calories from fats, almost all of which are saturated animal fats. Meats such as beef, pork, and lamb—which have very unbalanced nutritional profiles—are high in saturated fats, very high in calories, and completely lacking in fiber. This is also the case for poultry and eggs, which are two of the top ten allergenic foods. Many people do not even know that they have this allergy, since they may not experience overt symptoms immediately after eating them. These foods are also a source of cholesterol—a single egg contains a whopping 250 mg. Excessive consumption of meat, poultry, and eggs has been clinically linked to various cancers and conditions like diabetes, arthritis, and heart and artery disease. The chart below, which is based on statistics from forty countries, shows that rates of heart disease deaths and saturated fat intake are strongly correlated (*Circulation*, v. 88, 1993). In addition, as shown in *The China Study* by Dr. T. Colin Campbell, excessive animal protein consumption is associated with shorter lifespan and lower quality of life.

Unfortunately, meats, poultry, and eggs are ubiquitous in Western culture, which makes it difficult to avoid them. Nevertheless, these foods must be cut from your diet, including products that are "organic" and "free-range." You can still eat fish and other seafood in moderation, but they should account for no more than 10 percent of your diet. If you want to be healthy and enjoy a high quality of life, you should stop eating animal products.

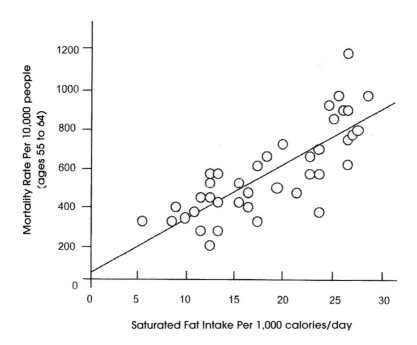

Relationship Between Saturated Fat Intake and Heart Disease Mortality

MILK AND DAIRY PRODUCTS

Milk and dairy products are just as bad, if not worse, than meat, poultry, and eggs. They are high in calories and saturated fats, lacking in fiber, and have an unbalanced ratio of vitamins and minerals. Another problem with dairy products is that they contain lactose, a sugar found in milk. Studies have shown that people lose the ability to digest lactose after childhood, when it ceases to be essential for survival. In fact, humans are the only mammals that continue to drink milk after infancy. In many cultures, though, milk and dairy products are not consumed. Africans and Asians in particular are notoriously lactose intolerant, a condition that is less obvious in Caucasians. Yogurt is even worse for you than milk, despite being commonly thought of as a "health food." This is because milk powder is added to yogurt as a thickening agent, doubling its lactose content. In addition, most dairy products contain casein, a type of protein that has been associated with cancer and other diseases.

Many people believe that substituting with organic or low-fat dairy foods is the answer, which couldn't be further from the truth. Even low-fat dairy products contain lactose and casein. The real solution is to cut all dairy products out of your diet and replace them with non-dairy milks, cheeses, and yogurts. Soy milk and soy cheeses are popular among vegetarians, and rice milk, almond milk, and oat milk are also good options. Keep trying different products until you find one that you like. You will quickly see a dramatic improvement in your health simply by removing milk and dairy products from your diet. Websites such as www.not milk.com can tell you more about the many reasons why eliminating dairy from your diet has such a positive impact on your health.

SUGAR

As mentioned already, the average American consumes approximately 160 pounds of sugar each year. This sugar habit has surely contributed to the high rates of insulin resistance, diabetes, and other blood sugar problems in the United States. Excessive sugar intake also raises blood lipid levels, which can lead to coronary heart disease. Even people who follow a vegetable-based diet can have health problems if they consume too much sugar. There is no such thing as a "good" form of sugar, whether it's artificial sugars like sucralose, or naturally occurring sugars like honey, syrup, agave, lo han, and molasses. Although fruit is generally thought of as being healthy, it contains large amounts of natural sugar and should be consumed only in moderation. Fruit should make up no more than 10 percent of your diet. Dried fruits, canned fruits, and fruit juices are even higher in sugar than raw fruit and should be avoided. Tropical fruits are very allergenic and tend to be better tolerated by those who live in tropical climates. Citrus fruits, such as lemons, oranges, grapefruits, and tangerines, rank among the top ten most allergenic food groups.

To reduce your consumption, start by cutting out dessert, which has become a bad habit common among the American population in particular. Replace cake and cookies with fresh raw fruit that is low in sugar. Macrobiotic cookbooks contain recipes for whole grain-based desserts, which are good temporary replacements as you transition to a dessert-free diet. Also eliminate processed foods that contain added sugars, especially high-fructose corn syrup, and all types of sweeteners, including ones that claim to be "natural," like stevia. Remember, sugar is sugar, regardless of its source.

WHOLE GRAINS

Whole grains are literally the "staff of life" and should be the foundation of your diet. Whole grains, which have been central to human nutrition for centuries, include brown rice, buckwheat, bulgur, barley, corn, rye, oats, millet, quinoa, spelt, teff, and whole wheat. Because they do not undergo processing, whole grains are rich in fiber and other important nutrients. In addition to their excellent nutritional profile, whole grains are low in fat and calories, as well as a source of high-quality protein. In recent years, there has been a lot of hype about "gluten intolerance" and celiac disease, a disorder characterized by the inability to digest *gluten,* a protein found in wheat. As a result, it has become popular to eat a "gluten-free diet," and cut out grains like wheat, rye, and barley. In reality, true gluten intolerance (celiac disease) is a very rare condition. Most people who think they are gluten intolerant are really suffering from irritable bowel syndrome (IBS) or a similar condition. Removing wheat from their diet is not going to help. In fact, cutting out grains has a negative impact—the average American diet already consists of less than 1 percent whole grains, and most bread products we eat are made from refined white flour that is stripped of all nutritional value.

Whole grains should account for about 50 percent of your diet. Boost your intake by eating whole-grain cereals or hot oatmeal, which is very low in calories and fat, for breakfast. One cup of cooked oats has only about 145 calories, 15 percent of which are from fat. You can also incorporate foods like polenta, a type of cornmeal, into your diet. A staple food in many countries, corn is very versatile and can be eaten fresh, frozen, as whole cornmeal (not degermed), or as a snack in the form of whole-grain corn chips. Corn grits, however, are almost always refined, so you should avoid them. For dinner, make barley soup or meals that include underutilized grains like buckwheat. Rye is not commonly eaten due to its strong flavor, but it makes for great-tasting bread. Quinoa, spelt, and teff tend to be more expensive than other grains, but they can add variety to your meals. And although most couscous is refined, there are some delicious whole-grain varieties available and sold in most supermarkets.

There are also more basic changes you can make to your daily diet in order to meet your requirement for whole grains, such as replacing white bread and pasta with whole-grain versions. Chain grocery stores now carry preservative-free, 100-percent whole-grain breads that have only about 70 calories per slice and contain about 8-percent protein. Two ounces of dry whole-wheat pasta (which makes about six ounces cooked) contains approximately 200 calories, only 5 percent of which are fat calories. Pay attention to nutrition labels, and buy products that list whole wheat as a main ingredient.

One of the most nutritious and versatile whole grains is brown rice, which is a staple food in many parts of the world. It is also one of the lowest allergenic foods. It's a good idea to buy 25- to 50-pound bags of short- or long-grain organic brown rice. One cup of cooked brown rice contains a mere 173 calories (only 5 percent of them from fat) and tons of nutrients. Add buckwheat to your brown rice dishes for flavor and variety, and buy brown rice pasta. Jasmine and basmati rice are also good choices, but you should save sweet rice for desserts.

BEANS

Beans should be a staple food in every diet. Like whole grains, beans are low in fat and calories, and loaded with fiber, protein, and an assortment of beneficial nutrients. Most bean varieties contain only about 120 calories (2 percent from fat) per cup, and a significant amount of protein—about 20 percent. There are many types of delicious beans available in your local grocery store, and ethnic and gourmet markets offer an even wider bean selection. Pinto beans, black beans, chickpeas, lentils, pink beans, kidney beans, adzuki beans, chili beans, lima beans, navy beans, northern beans, fava beans, mayocoba beans, and cannellini beans are just some of the varieties you will find.

Bean allergies, including soybean allergies, are rare. Soybeans cultivated today have high oil content, but very few people eat cooked dried soybeans anyway. A good recipe book will show you how to cook and prepare beans in versatile, flavorful, and delicious ways. Bean soups, bean dips, refried beans, bean sprouts, and bean spreads like hummus are all great options. You'll find that they taste as good as they are good for you. However, keep in mind that tofu, a bean product made from soybeans, is a heavily refined food that lacks nutrients.

VEGETABLES

Unlike most Asian populations (especially Chinese, Vietnamese, and Thai people), Americans generally do not eat a sufficient amount of vegetables, which form the basis of any good diet. Most vegetables have practically no fat, are very low in calories, and are loaded with fiber and nutrients like beta carotene, a compound with antioxidant properties (see page 118). They also contain substances called *lignans*, a group of antioxidants, and *sterols*, which can help lower lipid levels, among other health benefits.

Colorful vegetables, especially yellow and leafy green vegetables, are delicious and particularly good for you. However, vegetables from the nightshade family—a category that includes potatoes, tomatoes, eggplant, and peppers—should be avoided, as they contain toxic alkaloids like solanine. These alkaloids have been found to affect nerve-muscle function, digestive function, and joint function. Tomatoes, which were considered to be an ornamental, inedible toxic plant for centuries, contain tomatine, which is also harmful when eaten in excess. Nightshade vegetables should be consumed only in small amounts, if they are eaten at all.

It's important that you include the right vegetables in your diet. Learn how to cook fresh vegetables in various international styles, which will make your meals more diverse, appealing, and flavorful. There is an abundance of recipes available for Asian vegetable dishes. You can also eat sea vegetables, which are popular in Asian cuisine and include dulse, hizike, wakame, nori, and kombu. Eat these only on occasion, since they contain very high amounts of iodine. If you are overweight or obese, consider going on an all-vegetable (or vegetable soup) diet for one week to jumpstart weight loss and fill your body with nutrients.

SEAFOOD

If you don't want to eat a 100-percent vegetarian diet, seafood is a good addition. Evidence shows that vegetarians who eat seafood in moderation are just as healthy as pure vegetarians, or vegans. Seafood should account for no more than 10 percent of your diet. One 4-ounce portion of fish or shellfish per day is a good amount. Be sure to choose low-fat white fish, such as flounder, snapper, and sole, instead of fish that have higher fat content, like catfish, turbot, swordfish, Before introducing seafood to your regular diet, make sure that you do not have an allergy or sensitivity. Seafood allergies may go unnoticed because their symptoms can be mild.

NUTS

Although often recommended as healthy snacks to people who are trying to lose weight, nuts are actually very high in fat, very high in calories, and have an unbalanced nutritional profile. Raw nuts should be used only as garnish for dishes such as salads, which is common in Asian cuisine, and nut butters can be consumed in moderation. It's important to note that peanuts are tropical legumes, not nuts, and are very allergenic. It should also be mentioned that nuts are not related botanically. In other words, "tree nuts" like almonds, hazelnuts, pecans, and walnuts do not belong to the same species. Therefore, the term "tree nut allergy" is not only overly simplistic, but also inaccurate. There are no tree nut allergies.

FOLLOWING A NATURAL DIET

Throughout the last few decades, especially in recent years, dieting has become a huge industry in the United States. The growing rates of obesity and other weight-related health problems are at least partially to blame. It seems that there's a new fad diet every week, but never one that is actually effective or healthy. For example, the Atkins diet—one of the most popular diets in history—involves consuming meat and animal fat in excess, while cutting out sugars and carbohydrates, including nutritious whole grains like brown rice. This approach is based on the *glycemic index,* a scale that ranks foods based on how they affect blood sugar levels in the body. The glycemic index also inspired the ketogenic diet, the South Beach diet, the so-called Paleolithic diet, and various other low-carb regimens. However, this ranking system is wrong because it does not make a distinction between simple and complex carbohydrates. According to this scale, there is little, if any, difference between whole grains and the simple sugars found in other carbohydrates.

Other misleading fad diets include the Mediterranean diet, which includes large amounts of cheese, tomatoes, and olive oil, and the blood-type diet, which, as its name suggests, involves eating specific foods according to your blood type. However, it does not provide any real health benefits. People who follow raw-food diets suffer from poor nutrition when they consume too much sugar from fruit, fruit juice, and other sources of natural sugars like honey, molasses, and honey. The same is true for vegetarians and vegans, who may also consume large amounts of sugar due to diets high in fruit and simple sugars.

The popularity of fad diets has had a detrimental effect on our health, as they encourage people to unknowingly eat all the wrong foods. Even worse is that the unscientific concepts on which many of these diets are based are published in the medical literature. Many well-known nutritionists and authors of diet books are actually poor role models for long health and longevity, and give bad advice when it comes to healthy eating. Still, there are a few knowledgeable health professionals who provide truly helpful, effective guidance about nutrition and practice what they preach, which is just as important. See "Recommended Reading" on page 147 for a list of books that offer great nutritional advice.

The macrobiotic diet, which consists primarily of whole grains, is also a good option and strongly recommended if you have a chronic illness. Traditional Japanese macrobiotics as advocated by Michio Kushi and George Ohsawa is unnecessarily rigid, so follow the Americanized version instead. With certain diet and lifestyle restrictions removed, the macrobiotic diet is practical, varied, fun, and delicious. There are a number of published accounts from people who experienced huge improvements in their health by following the macrobiotic lifestyle. Books like *My Beautiful Life* (Mina Dobic), *Recalled By Life* (Anthony J. Sattilaro), and *Confessions of a Kamikaze Cowboy* (Dirk Benedict) recount how they used macrobiotics instead of allopathic medicine to treat "incurable" diseases like cancer.

So, with the abundance of conflicting and confusing information out there, how do you do you choose the right diet? How do you decide which approach to nutrition is the healthiest and most ideal? The simple answer is to look at the real-world results. Individuals who follow natural diets like macrobiotics have experienced real results, and there are plenty of books in which you can read their stories for yourself. Do not be fooled by fad diets, no matter how popular. Do your research and find out the facts.

CONCLUSION

Eating a natural diet not only means eating whole unprocessed foods, but also eating according to your genetics and environment. People who live in tropical climates, for instance, should eat foods like mangos, avocados, and papayas, which are indigenous to their climate and environment. Likewise, people who live in temperate climates should eat the foods available in their natural environments to which their bodies are accustomed. Nature always provides us with food in our environments that are proper to our genetics. The next time you consider starting the latest diet craze, take a natural approach instead. There are no quick fixes when it comes to your health, and when it comes to eating right, total lifestyle change is necessary.

15. Fasting

Dating back to ancient times, fasting—a practice in which you stop all food intake for a period of time and consume only water—is one of the most powerful healing methods available to us. Yet most people do not realize that fasting offers a wide range of health benefits that are not only physical, but also psychological, intellectual, emotional, and spiritual. The Western population, which tends to over-eat all the wrong foods, has the most to benefit from fasting. As you already know, Americans literally eat twice the number of calories that they need every day, and most of these calories come from unhealthy fats, sugar, and refined foods. Adopting a natural diet and fasting regularly helps to detoxify your body, ridding it of harmful substances, as well as change your eating habits and lessen your obsession with food. This chapter gives you the information you need to make fasting a part of your lifestyle so that you can optimize your well-being and quality of life.

WHAT IS FASTING?

Hippocrates once said, "Natural forces within us are the true healers of disease." This is the philosophical foundation of fasting. In general, fasting is a healing and cleansing practice in which an individual may abstain from all foods and liquids except water for a certain period of time. A fast, which can last anywhere from twenty-four hours to two weeks, can be used to detoxify the body, treat a specific medical condition, lose weight, or simply boost your overall health.

Fasting has been practiced for centuries. In most of the major religions—including Christianity, Islam, Judaism, Buddhism, Hinduism, Mormonism, and Native American spirituality—fasting is traditional method of observance. Fasting is mentioned repeatedly in both the Old and New Testaments of the Bible, and in cultures around the world, it has been used for hundreds of years to cure illness, clear the mind, and strengthen, revitalize, and cleanse the body. Today, holistic nutritionists and naturopathic doctors encourage people to fast in order to rid the body of harmful toxins taken in through unhealthy foods and the environment, as well as increase energy, improve immunity, and sleep better, among other benefits. Fasting can also be used as a preventive and therapeutic measure for various chronic diseases, from allergies to obesity.

Water fasts—abstaining from all foods and beverages except water—are the only true fasts. "Fasts" that eliminate certain foods are not real fasts, so they do not detoxify and repair the body to the same extent as water fasts. Moreover, juice fasts—consuming only fruit and vegetable juices for a specific period of time—are also not beneficial, since you end up consuming an excessive amount of sugar from the fruits being juiced. Water fasts may be difficult at first, but no other type of fast has a greater effect on your health.

THE BENEFITS OF FASTING

Fasting regularly will help you live both longer and better. Research has long shown that calorie restriction can help increase lifespan, slow the aging process, and reduce the risk of cancer, diabetes and insulin resistance, heart disease, and immune disorders, among other chronic diseases. The same is true for fasting. It also provides you with energy, relaxation, and mental and emotional clarity, as well as improved mood, resistance against disease, and weight loss. When you fast, your body does not have to expend energy breaking down and metabolizing food, allowing it to perform other actions like eliminating toxins, repairing cells, and removing wastes.

Natural health practitioners recommend fasting to treat a number of ailments, including the common cold, fever, flu, headaches, allergies, asthma, insomnia, skin problems, digestive conditions (such as constipation), fatigue, and obesity. Fasting also helps remove toxins and chemicals taken into the body through processed food consumption and the environment. In addition, fasting regularly can have a positive influence on individual eating habits and diet, which is particularly beneficial for those who typically follow a diet high in fat, sugar, and refined foods. Through fasting, you learn that hunger is more often a desire than an actual physical need, and that willpower is an illusion. Most of the time, "hunger" is not caused by a physical requirement for calories, but rather a desire to fulfill some emotional need. By fasting regularly, you will learn the difference between physical hunger and the desire to eat. Abstaining from food for a short period of time can actually be rejuvenating and transform the way you eat. But before taking this important step towards better health, you should have a clear understanding of how and when to fast.

HOW TO FAST

As already mentioned, the length of a fast can range from one day to two weeks. Of course, you should not start with a two-week fast if it's your first time. It's important to ease into the process gradually so that you do not experience any adverse side effects. Long fasts (one to two weeks) are generally intended to treat serious conditions, but can also be done for the purpose of general wellness. When fasting for this length of time, you should go to a spa or clinic to get the necessary psychological support, as well as a full physical evaluation. There are few fasting centers in the United States, but there are many spas and health clinics that can provide assistance. If you're simply looking to boost your overall health, one- to two-day fasts are sufficient and do not require supervision. However, people with conditions like diabetes and blood sugar disorders should not fast until they are well. Women who are nursing or pregnant should not fast for longer than one to two days.

To prepare your body for longer fasts, start by fasting for one day per week, from dinner to dinner, drinking only water. Eat an early dinner on Friday, for example, and do not eat again until dinnertime on Saturday. You can also choose to fast from breakfast to breakfast, or from lunch to lunch, if that works better for you. If fasting for twenty-four hours is too difficult at first, you can gradually acclimate your body by skipping breakfast once a week for four weeks. After four weeks, eliminate lunch as well. When you can go without breakfast and lunch, you will be doing a one-day fast. Fast for one day once every four weeks, and fast for two days once a month. If you are unable to fast on your usual day of the week for whatever reason, fast the day before or the day after instead. Vacations are a great time to fast.

During one-day fasts, continue to take the recommended supplements—including vitamins, minerals, and other nutrients—listed in Chapters 16 and 17 (see pages 117 and 131), as well as any bioidentical hormones you are using. When fasting for two days or longer, you need to take only the necessary hormone supplements, along with acidophilus, FOS, and L-glutamine (see pages 118, 120, and 121), which are even more effective when you do not have any food in your system. All the other supplements are optional.

While it's important to get plenty of rest while fasting, exercise is also essential. A low-impact activity like walking is the best form of exercise to do during a fast, since it does not require you to expend significant amounts of energy. Resistance exercise can be done as well if you are not fatigued. Some people feel weak during a fast, but others have more energy and endurance. Listen to your body.

It's important to note that longer fasts may cause temporary side effects—such as fatigue, headaches, general weakness, or dizziness upon standing up—which usually affect people the most on the third day. Remember that side effects are common and likely to go away on their own. If you experience more intense symptoms of any kind, stop the fast immediately and have a bowl of hot soup. Should side effects continue or worsen, it is usually a sign of an underlying medical condition, such as diabetes or hypoglycemia, which may need to be assessed.

You can break short (one- and two-day) fasts simply by eating a small meal of natural foods. Long fasts, however, should not be ended abruptly. Start by having a bowl of healthy soup, wait thirty minutes, and then eat a small meal of all whole natural foods.

CONCLUSION

Enhancing the quality of your life is just as important as increasing the length of your life, and you can achieve both of these goals when you fast. Fasting is one of the Seven Steps to Natural Health (see page 143), and a healing practice that will revitalize your body, drastically improve your eating habits, and help you attain optimal wellness. Fasting also maximizes the benefits of a natural whole-foods diet. It is the most powerful healing method available to us.

Of course, the more information you have about fasting, the more likely you will be to do it. A variety of great books on the topic are listed under "Recommended Reading" on page 147. You should also consider participating in Young Again's two-day international fasts, which are held on the last weekend of every month, from Thursday to Saturday. Additional information and fasting schedules are available at www.YoungAgain.org. Here you will also find several articles on fasting, such as "Do a Five Day Fast in 72 Hours." If it's difficult for you to go two days without food at first, just work up to it gradually. Although the idea of consuming nothing but water for two days may be intimidating at first, it really is easier than you think, and every month it will be a little easier. You will feel and actually *be* healthier as a result.

16. Essential Vitamins and Other Nutrients

onsidering the vast selection of nutritional supplements on the market today, choosing the ones that are actually beneficial can be overwhelming and confusing. Most of what you read and hear about some products is simply hype, and not at all based on science. The supplement industry is just as interested in making a profit as any other—making people healthier is not exactly their number one priority. Still, there are a number of natural, safe, inexpensive, and proven supplements that you can take to be healthier, feel better, and live longer—without prescription drugs. This chapter lists specific vitamins and other nutrients that are essential for good health, providing dosage guidelines and explanations of how they work in your body. While many of these supplements should be permanent additions to your diet, remember that they are not intended to take the place of nutritious natural foods and a healthy lifestyle.

ENDOGENEOUS SUPPLEMENTS

Endogenous supplements are naturally present in your body and found in many foods. You should take these supplements in the appropriate and recommended amounts to enhance your health. These substances can and should be used permanently, especially if you are over forty years of age. If you are under forty, take only the supplements that are starred with an asterisk [*]—acidophilus, beta glucan, flaxseed oil, FOS, L-glutamine (optional), and vitamins D and E—as well as a multivitamin and complete mineral supplement, which is discussed more in Chapter 17 (see page 131).

Acetyl-L-Carnitine (ALC)

Acetyl-L-carnitine (ALC), an amino acid used to produce energy in the body, is the preferred form of L-carnitine, as it is more easily absorbed. ALC has powerful antioxidant properties that promote proper brain metabolism and memory. There are a number of studies showing that ALC also helps to maintain cognitive abilities in elderly people. Other studies suggest that ALC may be beneficial for some heart conditions and mental disorders. The supplement is most effective when used with phosphatidylserine (see page 122) and pregnenolone (see page 33).

Recommended Dosage: 500 to 1,000 mg per day.

Acidophilus*

Acidophilus (*Lactobacillus acidophilus*) belongs to a group known as probiotics, "good bacteria" that help to maintain the health of the intestinal tract and aid digestion. Human studies have shown that acidophilus is also effective for bacterial vaginosis, a common infection. When taking acidophilus supplements, use only reputable brands that contain about eight different acidophilus strains, as well as at least 6 billion colony-forming units (CFUs) per capsule. Buy only refrigerated acidophilus, and keep the supplement in your refrigerator to keep it from going bad. Use along with fructooligosaccarides (FOS) and L-glutamine supplements (see pages 120 and 121).

Recommended Dosage: 6 billion CFUs per day.

Beta Carotene

This compound belongs to the *carotenoid* family, a group of pigmented substances present in many fruits and vegetables, including apricots, carrots, spinach, squash, and sweet potatoes. *Beta carotene* is the precursor to vitamin A, which means that it can be converted into the vitamin and its analogs, such as retinol and retinoic acid. It is also one of the most powerful antioxidants, so a deficiency can lead to free radical damage in the body, in turn causing inflammation, among other problems. Beta-carotene deficiency is also linked to weakened immunity and increased risk of cancer and heart disease.

Recommended Dosage: 10,000 international units (IU) per day.

Beta Glucan*

A polysaccharide found in the cells walls of bacteria, fungi, yeasts, *beta glucan* is the most powerful immune enhancer known to science. Beta glucan, which is also contained in oats and barley, has been shown to have a positive effect on blood sugar dysmetabolism, cancer, high cholesterol, allergies, and common infections, among other medical conditions. It has also been shown to benefit heart health, as it helps to lower cholesterol and triglycerides (see page 87). This is a basic supplement that should be used by everyone, regardless of your age or health. If you eat oatmeal or barley regularly, you do not need to take beta glucan in supplement form.

Recommended Dosage: 200 to 400 mg per day.

Beta-Sitosterol

Every vegetable you eat contains *beta-sitoserol*, a plant sterol that supports breast and uterine health, and helps reduce cholesterol levels. The average American adult takes in an estimated 300 mg per day, while vegetarians eat double that amount and suffer from fewer health problems. When taking beta-sitosterol supplements, make sure you use a product that contains mixed sterols for the most benefits. Check the ingredients list on the label.

Recommended Dosage: 300 to 600 mg per day.

Coenzyme Q_{10} (CoQ_{10})

A powerful antioxidant normally produced by the body, *coenzyme Q_{10}*, or CoQ_{10}, is necessary for proper cell function. Low levels are found in people with medical conditions such as diabetes, cancer, and heart problems. CoQ_{10} is a vital element in any supplement program. Be careful not to buy expensive products claiming to have "special delivery systems," which are completely unnecessary. Also, do not use ubiquinol, which is very unstable, has no shelf life, and is not even real CoQ_{10}. Use real Japanese ubiquinone for the most benefits.

Recommended Dosage: 100 mg per day. Elderly people and individuals with certain medical conditions should take 200 mg per day.

Diindolylmethane (DIM)

Diindolylmethane (DIM) is produced during the digestion of indole-3-carbinol, a substance found in vegetables like Brussels sprouts, broccoli, cabbage, and kale. In addition to having potential anti-cancer properties, DIM acts as an anti-inflammatory agent and is essential for estrogen metabolism and balance. There is no need for you to take this substance if your estradiol and estrone levels are in low-normal ranges and your estriol level is in the high-normal range. Do not buy products that claim to have "special delivery systems." Since DIM is oil-soluble, it should be taken with food or flaxseed oil for better absorption.

Recommended Dosage: 200 mg per day.

Flaxseed Oil*

Extracted from the seeds of the flax plant, *flaxseed oil* is rich in omega-3 fatty acids, which act as antioxidants in the body. Flaxseed oil is a better source of omega-3s than fish oil, as it contains lignans (beneficial phytonutrients) and no arachidonic acid—an unhealthy fat found in red meats, organ meats, and egg yolks. There is an overwhelming amount of research on the benefits of omega-3 supplementation for blood sugar metabolism, cardiovascular health, and blood lipid levels. The supplement, which contains a mere nine fat calories per capsule, should be taken by everyone, regardless of age. Do not buy unrefrigerated flax oil, as it easily oxidizes, and keep the product refrigerated.

Recommended Dosage: 1,000 to 2,000 mg per day, or $^1/_2$ tsp of bulk flaxseed oil.

Folic Acid

Folic acid, or *folate*, is a water-soluble B vitamin that plays a vital role in heart health and enables the development of healthy cells. Folic acid is a female-specific vitamin, so women of child-bearing age should consume a sufficient amount of folic acid in order to maintain good health and prevent birth defects. Folic acid is naturally found in many foods, such as leafy green vegetables, legumes, dried beans, nuts, yeast, some fruits, and enriched breads, cereals, and pastas. Folic acid supplements can be used to correct a deficiency, but it cannot replace a healthy diet rich in B vitamins.

Recommended Dosage: 800 mcg per day.

Fructooligosaccharides (FOS)*

Belonging to a group known as prebiotics, *fructooligosaccharides* (FOS), or *inulin,* are non-digestible sugars that improve your intestinal flora—"good" bacteria. This biological activity is highly beneficial, since poor digestive health is an epidemic in Western countries due to factors like an unhealthy diet and inactive lifestyle. In addition to promoting gastrointestinal and colon health, FOS has been reported to help treat yeast infections. Significant amounts are not found in your food, so supplementation is vital. Use

FOS supplements in combination with acidophilus and L-glutamine (see pages 118 and below) for the most benefits.

Recommended Dosage: 750 to 1,500 mg per day.

Glucosamine

This naturally occurring compound is a basic building block of cartilage and connective tissue, which is why it is beneficial for bone and joint conditions. *Glucosamine* needs co-factors in order to be effective. This means that it should be taken alongside a complete supply of minerals, as well as flaxseed oil and vitamin D (see pages 120 and 124). Glucosamine supplements are essential, especially when joint or bone problems are present.

Recommended Dosage: 500 to 1,000 mg per day.

Lecithin

Extracted from foods like soybeans, *lecithin* is an essential healthy fat that can be used for lowering cholesterol, as well as supporting good brain metabolism. Lecithin may also be effective against gallbladder disease, liver disease, anxiety, and eczema, a skin condition. This supplement is optional, but anyone who is at risk for cardiovascular problems or suffers from heart disease should take it. Use softgel capsules.

Recommended Dosage: 1,200 mg per day.

L-glutamine*

L-glutamine, or glutamine, is an amino acid and prebiotic. Numerous studies support its use against intestinal conditions, particularly when taken in combination with acidophilus and FOS (see pages 118 and 120). L-glutamine causes human growth hormone (HGH) hormone levels to spike, but this fluctuation is only temporary. The supplement is inexpensive and can be purchased as tablets or in bulk. It's a good idea for people under forty years of age to take L-glutamine; for people over forty, this supplement is vital.

Recommended Dosage: 1,000 mg per day for long-term use; 1 to 2 tbsp of the powder per day for one year to strengthen digestion.

Lipoic Acid

An antioxidant made naturally by the body, *lipoic acid*—also known as alpha-lipoic acid—is found in all of your cells and helps convert glucose into energy. As a supplement, lipoic acid helps normalize blood sugar and insulin levels, as well as maintain good cardiovascular health. Studies suggest that it may also protect brain and nerve tissue. Do not use R-lipoic acid, which is overpriced and unnecessary. All clinical studies use regular lipoic acid. Since this substance is not found in food sources, supplementation is highly beneficial.

Recommended Dosage: 400 mg per day.

N-Acetyl Cysteine (NAC)

N-acetyl cysteine, or NAC, is an antioxidant derived from the amino acid L-cysteine that has multiple medicinal uses. One of its most important benefits is its ability to raise levels of glutathione, one of the two major antioxidant enzymes in the body, which decreases as you age. In fact, NAC is better for raising glutathione levels than glutathione itself, which is ineffective when taken orally.

Recommended Dosage: 600 mg per day.

Phosphatidylserine (PS)

Related to lecithin (see page 121), *phosphatidylserine* (PS) is a chemical naturally found in human brain tissue, as well as some foods, including white beans and soybeans. PS was made available to the public only in recent years thanks to the publication of more studies showing its benefits for brain function and memory. PS may also help lower cholesterol and triglyceride levels. It is most effective when used in combination with pregnenolone (see page 33) and acetyl-L-carnitine (see page 118). Take the supplement as a soft gel capsule.

Recommended Dosage: 100 mg per day.

Quercetin

This compound is a plant pigment belonging to the antioxidant *flavonoid* family. Quercetin also has anti-inflammatory and antihistamine properties, making it effective against allergies, heart disease, and cancer. In people with hypertension, quercetin may help lower cholesterol levels and reduce blood pressure. Dietary sources of quercetin include apples, apricots, blueberries, broccoli, buckwheat, cherries, cranberries, currants, kale, grapes, and onions. Quercetin supplements are inexpensive, and can be found in pill or capsule form.

Recommended Dosage: 100 mg per day.

Soy Isoflavones

Isoflavones are naturally occurring compounds that have antioxidant properties and other beneficial effects. The primary isoflavones in soy are genistein and daidzein, which support hormone balance, lower lipid levels and blood pressure, help prevent osteoporosis, and alleviate PMS and menopause symptoms. These isoflavones are found in soy foods—such as miso, seitan, tempeh, soybeans, soy flour, and soy milk— which have been staple foods in many cultures (particularly Asian) for centuries. However, in the United States and other Western countries, the best way to get isoflavones is to use supplements, since most people do not eat an adequate amount of soy foods. There is an overwhelming amount of published research on the benefits of soy isoflavones; the Asian population alone sufficiently demonstrates the impact of soy isoflavones on overall health and longevity. Okinawans consume the most soy and have the longest lifespan out of any other population in the world. When supplementing with soy isoflavones, be sure to use a product that contains both genistein and daidzein.

Recommended Dosage: 40 mg per day.

Vitamin B_6

This female-specific, water-soluble vitamin helps the body produce energy and is needed for nervous system function. Studies suggest that the vitamin supports proper vision and mental health. B_6 is present in many foods, including grains, legumes, fish, and some vegetables, such as carrots, peas, and spinach. Women can also benefit from having adequate B_6 in their diet, as it may aid in relieving PMS symptoms. The recommended daily allowance (RDA) is about 2 mg per day, but consuming 10 mg per day results in more benefits. Although some short-term studies have used large doses of 50 mg or more, megadoses are always contraindicated.

Recommended Dosage: 2 to 10 mg per day.

Vitamin B_{12}

Another water-soluble B-complex vitamin, B_{12} plays a key role in human metabolism, as well as brain and nervous system function. Vitamin B_{12} is usually taken in through the diet, but supplements can be helpful if you have certain health problems. Take methylcobalamin, which is the most bioavailable form of B_{12} and involved in human metabolism. Regular vitamin B_{12} is poorly absorbed when taken orally.

Recommended Dosage: 1 mg per day.

Vitamin C

In addition to acting as an antioxidant, this essential vitamin protects against conditions ranging from cancer to the common cold. It also helps decrease blood sugar, repair tissues, and boost the immune system. Despite these benefits, vitamin C is a very overrated vitamin. It is abundant mainly in citrus fruits (papaya, oranges, and grapefruit, for example), which are meant to be eaten by people who live in tropical—not temperate—climates. Megadoses of vitamin C will acidify your blood, which can cause serious problems over time. The recommended daily allowance—90 mg per day for men, and 75 mg per day for women who are not pregnant or nursing—is sufficient, but you can take up to 250 mg per day for specific health issues.

Recommended Dosage: 75 to 250 mg per day.

Vitamin D*

Vitamin D is actually an oil-soluble hormone, not a vitamin. Vitamin D_3 is the form used by the human body and taken as a supplement. Almost no vitamin D is found in food; exposure to sunlight is the only real source. Research has shown that vitamin D helps maintain strong bones and protect against high blood pressure, osteoporosis, certain cancers, and various autoimmune diseases. Unfortunately, many people are deficient in vitamin D, so supplementation is crucial and highly beneficial. In addition to the 400 IU you'll find in most multivitamin supplements, take another 400 IU of vitamin D if you are not in the sun regularly. However, dosage amounts should never exceed 1,200 IU per day.

Recommended Dosage: 400 to 1,200 IU per day.

Vitamin E*

The name "vitamin E" actually refers to eight fat-soluble antioxidant compounds that are categorized as either *tocopherols* or *tocotrienols*. These antioxidants are naturally present in a variety of foods, especially leafy green vegetables and whole grains, which, as you already know, are lacking in the standard Western diet. Vitamin E has numerous health benefits, particularly for the arteries and heart. It can help lower blood pressure, reduce the risk of heart attack and chest pain (angina), and prevent hardened and blocked arteries. Always buy vitamin E supplements that contain natural mixed tocopherols, which is the most natural and complete form. Do not take synthetic d-alpha tocopherol supplements.

Recommended Dosage: 200 IU per day, or 400 IU every other day.

Multivitamins

In addition to these supplements, you definitely want to take a multivitamin. A multivitamin is a basic component of a healthy lifestyle program and should contain all thirteen essential vitamins—A, C, D, E, folate, B_6, B_{12}, thiamine, riboflavin, niacin, pantothenic acid, biotin, and K_1. Despite claims to the contrary, most multivitamin supplements are synthesized by necessity. It is better to buy a vitamins-only formula and take a separate complete mineral supplement. (See Chapter 17 on page 131 for a listing of essential minerals.) Choose a multivitamin that contains vitamin B_{12} in the form of methylcobalamin, since regular B_{12} cannot be absorbed when taken orally. Women should take extra vitamin B_6 and folic acid. It is somewhat difficult to find a mineral supplement that contains all the essential minerals, which are discussed in the next chapter. Most formulas contain ten elements at most and use "fillers" like phosphorus, potassium, and sulfur. Keep this in mind so that you choose a quality supplement.

EXOGENOUS SUPPLEMENTS

Unlike the supplements listed on the previous pages, the supplements described in this section are *exogeneous*—they are not found in dietary sources or made naturally by the body. They are also effective *only* in the short-term and, therefore, should be taken for no longer than six to twelve months. Be aware that exogeneous supplements do not work for everyone; some people may even be allergic. The agents listed in the pages that follow can help treat certain medical conditions and even facilitate weight loss. Still, keep in mind that they are optional and not essential for maintaining your overall health.

Aloe Vera

For thousands of years, gel from the leaves of the *Aloe vera* plant has been used topically to treat skin conditions such as wounds, infections, and burns. It is also a time-proven remedy for poor digestion and ulcers, and it helps immune function, liver function, digestive issues, and blood sugar regulation. Use a product that contains a 200:1 concentrate of pure aloe vera.

Recommended Dosage: Two 100-mg capsules per day.

Citrus Pectin

Derived from the pulp or peel of citrus fruits, *citrus pectin* helps digestion, as well as lowers cholesterol and triglycerides levels safely and naturally.

Do not buy modified citrus pectin, which is overpriced and completely unnecessary. Plain citrus pectin is fully absorbable and does not need to be "modified." Apple pectin is also an acceptable supplement to use.

Recommended Dosage: 3,000 mg per day.

Curcumin

Curcumin is the principal ingredient of turmeric, a popular Indian spice. In addition to its antioxidant properties, curcumin can improve digestive problems and help regulate blood glucose levels. The beneficial effects of curcumin have been demonstrated in numerous studies.

Recommended Dosage: 500 mg per day.

Ellagic Acid

This naturally occurring chemical is found primarily in walnut hulls. Studies have shown that *ellagic acid* acts as an antioxidant and has anti-cancer properties.

Recommended Dosage: 100 mg per day.

Green Tea

Made from the leaves of the *Camellia sinensis* plant, green tea has numerous health-giving properties due to its high concentration of powerful antioxidants known as polyphenols. Results of numerous studies have indicated that green tea is effective for preventing and treating high cholesterol, as well as various types of cancer, diabetes, liver disease, atherosclerosis (the hardening and narrowing of arteries). Drinking green tea regularly also promotes weight loss. To supplement with green tea, always use a decaffeinated extract.

Recommended Dosage: 200 mg per day.

Milk Thistle

This herb has been used for medicinal purposes for thousands of years. Its active ingredient is silymarin, which is extracted from the plant's seeds. *Milk thistle* is an effective liver rejuvenator and may be used to treat gallbladder disorders. You will receive the most benefits from this supplement if you take it along with TMG (see page 127) while following a low-fat diet. Look for a supplement that contains 40 percent silymarin.

Recommended Dosage: 400 mg per day.

Sodium Alginate

A natural seaweed extract, *sodium alginate* helps remove heavy metals like mercury, lead, and cadmium from your blood. The presence of these metals in the blood is often due to environmental factors, and they act as poisons in the body as they build up over time. Sodium alginate is far more effective than chelation therapy (both oral and injected), which does not work and is not a natural health practice.

Recommended Dosage: 3 g per day.

Trimethylglycine (TMG)

Trimethylglycine, or TMG, is a naturally occurring compound found in plants, and the most powerful liver supplement known to science. It also has a positive effect on blood sugar disorders, and can be used long-term to lower homocysteine levels and promote heart health.

Recommended Dosage: If using temporarily, take 3 g per day. For long-term use, take 1 g daily.

Remember, even though supplements are designed to enhance health and nutrition, substances often affect people in different ways. If you have a health condition, speak to a health-care professional before beginning a supplement regimen.

UNPROVEN SUPPLEMENTS

While the supplements highlighted in the first two sections of this chapter are based on numerous studies, there are many other products touted by the natural health industry that are not supported by science. Supplements for which there is no clinical evidence include:

- AHCC (Active Hexose Correlated Compound)
- Arginine
- Astaxanhin
- Bee pollen and other bee products
- Breast enhancers
- Coral calcium
- Chorella
- Chrondroitin
- Chrysin
- Coconut oil
- Colloidal minerals
- Colostrum
- Conjugated linolenic acid (CLA)
- Deer antler velvet

- Epimedium ("horny goat weed") and other libido/ virility enhancers
- 5-HTP
- Glyconutrients
- Grapefruit seed extract
- Graviola
- Gymnema
- Homeopathic remedies
- Hoodia
- Human growth hormone (HGH) supplements available over the counter
- Hyaluronic acid
- Lycopene
- Maca root
- Mangosteen products

- MGN-3
- Modified citrus pectin
- Noni juice
- Olive leaf
- Policosanol
- Pomegranate products
- Red yeast rice
- Resveratrol
- Saw palmetto
- 7-keto DHEA
- Spirulina
- Superoxide dismutase (SOD), oral supplements
- Tongkat ali
- Tribulus terrestris
- Whey protein

There are many more supplements that are not supported by science. Be sure to do thorough research to ensure you choose products that are safe, effective, and worth your money.

CONCLUSION

Although the supplements in this chapter are beneficial and even vital to your health, remember that no amount of supplementation is truly going to help you unless you are eating and living well. A low-fat, low-sugar diet based on whole grains is the foundation of good natural health. Remember, if you are under forty years of age, you only need to take acidophilus, beta glucan, flaxseed oil, FOS, vitamins D and E, and a complete vitamin and mineral supplement. But if you are forty or older, take all the essential supplements, plus supplements you need for any specific health issues you have. Spending your money on these scientifically backed supplements right now will save you a significant amount of money trying to treat serious medical conditions in the future.

ESSENTIAL VITAMINS AND NUTRITIONAL SUPPLEMENTS

Supplement	Optimal Daily Intake	Considerations
Acetyl-L-carnitine (ALC)	500 to 1,000 mg	Most effective when used in combination with pregnenolone and phosphatidylserine (PS).
Acidophilus*	6 billion colony-forming units (CFUs)	Keep refrigerated. Use with fructooligo-saccharides (FOS) and L-glutamine.
Beta carotene	10,000 international units (IU)	This powerful antioxidant can be used to reduce inflammation and boost immunity.
Beta glucan*	200 to 400 mg	Eating oatmeal or barley regularly is an acceptable alternative to taking supplements.
Beta-sitosterol	300 to 600 mg	Use a product that contains mixed sterols.
Coenzyme Q_{10} (CoQ_{10})	100 mg; 200 mg for elderly people and individuals with certain medical conditions	Do not use ubiquinol or products that claim to have special delivery systems. Real Japanese ubiquinone provides the most benefits.
Diindolylmethane (DIM)	200 mg	Do not use products claiming to have special delivery systems. Take with food or flaxseed oil for better absorption.
Flaxseed oil*	1,000 to 2,000 mg, or $1/2$ tsp of bulk flaxseed oil	Do not use unrefrigerated products.
Folic acid	800 mcg	Folic acid supplements should not be used as a replacement for a diet rich in B vitamins.
Fructooligo-saccharides (FOS)*	750 to 1,500 mg	Use in combination with acidophilus and L-glutamine for the most benefits.
Glucosamine	500 to 1,000 mg	Should be taken with a complete mineral supplement, flaxseed oil, and vitamin D.
Lecithin	1,200 mg	Especially recommended for people who have cardiovascular problems or a history of heart disease.
L-glutamine*	1,000 mg per day for long-term use; for digestion, 1 to 2 tbsp per day for one year	Causes a temporary spike in human growth hormone (HGH) levels. Most effective when used in combination with acidophilus and FOS.
Lipoic acid	400 mg	Supplementing with lipoic acid is highly beneficial, since the substance is not found in foods. Do not use R-lipoic acid.
N-acetyl cysteine (NAC)	600 mg	Helps raise levels of glutathione, a powerful antioxidant.
Phosphatidylserine (PS)	100 mg	Most effective when used with pregnenolone and acetyl-L-carnitine (ALC).

*Supplements marked by an asterisk (*) should be taken by women of all ages. All other supplements need only be taken by women who are over forty years of age.

Supplement	Optimal Daily Intake	Considerations
Quercetin	100 mg	Found in many foods like apricots, blueberries, and kale, quercetin is effective against allergies, cancer, and heart disease.
Soy isoflavones	40 mg	Use a supplement that contains both genistein and daidzein, which are the primary isoflavones in soy.
Vitamin B_6	2 to 10 mg	Do not take in large doses. B_6 is also present in many foods such as leafy greens, legumes, and fish.
Vitamin B_{12}	1 mg	Poorly absorbed when taken orally. Use supplements that contain B_{12} in the form of methylcobalamin, which is the most potent.
Vitamin C	75 to 250 mg	Do not take in megadoses, as excessive amounts acidify the blood.
Vitamin D*	400 to 1,200 mg	If you are not in the sun regularly, take an additional 400 mg per day. Never take more than 1,200 mg daily.
Vitamin E*	200 IU or 400 IU every other day	Use supplements that contain natural mixed tocopherols. Do not take synthetic d-alpha tocopherol supplements.

OPTIONAL NUTRITIONAL SUPPLEMENTS

Supplement	Optimal Daily Intake	Considerations
Aloe vera	200 mg	Use a product that contains a 200:1 concentrate of pure aloe vera.
Citrus pectin	3,000 mg	Do not buy modified citrus pectin, which is very overpriced. Apple pectin is an acceptable and equally beneficial alternative.
Curcumin	500 mg	Principal ingredient of turmeric, an Indian spice. Curcumin acts as an antioxidant, regulates blood sugar, and improves digestion.
Ellagic acid	100 mg	Antioxidant with anti-cancer properties.
Green tea	200 mg	Use a decaffeinated extract.
Milk thistle	400 mg	For the most benefits from this supplement, take with trimethylglycine (TMG) and follow a low-fat diet.
Sodium alginate	3 g	More effective than chelation therapy for removing heavy metals from the body.
Trimethylglycine (TMG)	3 g; for long-term use, 1 g	Enhances liver function, promotes heart health, and aids in blood sugar management.

17. Essential Minerals

No matter how well you eat, how many supplements you take, or how often you exercise, you will never attain optimal health unless you have sufficient levels of all the minerals you need. *Minerals* are inorganic elements found in the soil and water that are required for proper nutrition. Some minerals, such as iron, are needed in significant amounts, while others—*trace* and *ultratrace elements*—are needed in very small quantities. Because the body does not naturally produce minerals, you must acquire them through dietary sources. However, since the Western diet is very low in minerals, supplementation is the only way to ensure that you maintain adequate levels.

Only a handful of minerals—for example, calcium, copper, iodine, magnesium, and zinc—have established recommended daily allowances (RDAs), but there are at least twenty elements that are vital for human nutrition. Minerals work synergistically in the body, which means that you need sufficient amounts of all of them. This chapter serves as an overview of the most important minerals and their bioavailable supplement forms, many of which are inexpensive salts (like zinc sulfate) or *chelates*—minerals bound in a way that makes them more easily digested. Information about buying minerals is also provided to help you choose quality products and steer clear of worthless supplements on the market.

BORON

Boron is the most overlooked essential mineral. The research on boron is overwhelming, yet most people are seriously deficient. It is necessary for bone and cartilage metabolism, hormone metabolism (especially testosterone), reproduction and pregnancy, athletic performance, countless enzyme reactions, vitamin D metabolism, brain function and cognition, blood metabolism, immune function, and many other important health factors. Boron has also been shown to be important to cardiovascular health, as it positively affects cholesterol levels. A deficiency of boron can contribute to high blood pressure.

Study after study has shown that Americans eat only about 1 mg of boron a day, with vegetarians getting the most. Because modern farming methods have made our soils boron-deficient, you cannot rely on whole grains, beans, vegetables, and fruits to consistently supply it. Most mineral formulas do not contain boron. Boric acid and boric citrate are good forms to take. There is no RDA, so find a product that contains 3 mg.

Recommended Dosage: 3 mg per day.

CALCIUM

Although *calcium* is needed to maintain bone strength and density, its overall importance is greatly overstated. The official RDA is a staggering 1,000 mg per day. This number is unnecessarily high, clinically unsupported, and can be achieved only by consuming excessive amounts of dairy products, which is simply unhealthy. As mentioned in Chapter 9 (see page 73), dairy products contain lactose, which most human beings are unable to digest efficiently, and casein, a protein that has been linked to a number of diseases. Americans eat more dairy than any other population in the world, but are falsely led to believe that they are deficient in calcium due to high rates of osteoporosis, arthritis, and other bone and joint diseases. This is caused not by inadequate dietary intake of calcium but by inadequate calcium absorption, which depends on having sufficient amounts of specific minerals, omega-3 fatty acids, progesterone, and testosterone. In other words, calcium needs "helpers" in order to carry out functions like forming bone cells and maintaining bone strength.

Instead of trying to take in an unnecessary 1,000 mg through dairy products, eat a varied diet of whole natural foods like whole grains, green leafy vegetables, most beans, sprouts, carrots, soy foods, and seafood. This wholesome diet will supply you with about 250 mg of calcium from dietary sources, which is sufficient. Take an additional 250 mg in supplement form for a total of 500 mg of calcium per day. Calcium citrate and calcium carbonate are both effective.

Recommended Dosage: 500 mg per day (250 mg from food sources and 250 mg from supplements).

CESIUM

Although discovered in 1860, *cesium* was acknowledged as an essential ultratrace element only recently. Studies have shown that there is a significant amount of cesium in our blood, and research continues to find more foods that contain the mineral. Common vegetables, such as Brussels sprouts, cabbage, onions, and peas, all have meaningful amounts of cesium. Every year, there are more studies about the role of cesium in human nutrition, so it's likely you'll hear more about this ultratrace element in the future. Cesium is almost never found in mineral formulas, so be sure to find one that does. Because large doses are toxic, do not take more than 100 mcg per day, which is a reasonable and safe dosage.

Recommended Dosage: 100 mcg per day.

CHROMIUM

Chromium is an essential mineral that helps to regulate insulin and blood sugar levels. An estimated 90 percent of Americans are deficient in chromium, which is found mainly in whole grains and cereals, as well as lean meats, brewer's yeast, and some spices. Pregnant women, vigorous exercisers, and the elderly often have low chromium levels. Taking in a sufficient amount of chromium has been shown to have a positive effect on cholesterol, triglycerides, and blood sugar, as well as to lower the risk of diseases like heart disease and diabetes. You can take chromium in the form of chelates, which are inexpensive and easily absorbed by the body. Chromium is also found in most complete mineral formulas. Do not listen to advertisements claiming that a certain patented form is the "best" or "only" form of chromium that works. This mineral must be in your supplement program, but to avoid toxicity, do not to take more than 400 mcg per day, which is the maximum recommended dose.

Recommended Dosage: 120 to 400 mcg per day.

COBALT

Cobalt is an overlooked element even though it is the basic building block of vitamin B_{12}. Humans cannot synthesize vitamin B_{12} without a sufficient amount of available cobalt. Good food sources of this trace mineral include fish, leafy green vegetables, nuts, and oats, but supplements may be necessary to meet your daily requirement. Oral forms of vitamin B_{12} are not easily absorbed by the body, so you should take the vitamin in the form of methylcobalamin. Studies indicate that humans should take in 25 mcg of cobalt per day, yet few people get this amount. It is possible to find a mineral formula that contains 25 mcg of cobalt or more.

Recommended Dosage: 25 mcg per day.

COPPER

Copper is a trace mineral that has a variety of important functions in the body. It is involved in the production of red blood cells, and helps to keep your blood vessels, immune system, nerves, and bones healthy. About 150 mg of copper is naturally present in the body, but more should be taken in through food sources like whole grains, beans, nuts, and some types of seafood. Although the official RDA is 2 mg, most Americans consume only half of this amount. You can take copper citrate, oxide, or gluconate, which are bioavailable and inexpensive supplement forms. Do not take large amounts of copper; dosages over 15 mg per day can produce toxic effects.

Recommended Dosage: 2 mg per day.

GALLIUM

Gallium is an important but often ignored ultratrace element. The earth's crust has an amazing 10 milligrams of gallium per kilogram (kg). Studies of human blood, as well as many foods, have shown that gallium is central to nutrition. Despite its presence in every bodily organ, most people are deficient in gallium. Although you need about 100 mcg per day, a Japanese study found that most people consume only 12 mcg daily. The book *Advances in Micronutrient Research* (1996) provides good evidence for the value of gallium, but more research on its benefits is needed. Gallium nitrate is the best supplement form.

Recommended Dosage: 100 mcg per day.

GERMANIUM

Germanium is almost never found in mineral formulas, and there is no recommended daily allowance. However, an impressive review of several studies on germanium, complete with seventy-two references, was published in the journal *Medical Hypothesis*. The review found that germanium is beneficial to human nutrition when taken in doses of 100 mcg per day. Much larger doses have been irresponsibly recommended, but you should not exceed 100 mcg daily. Take germanium in the form of chelates or germanium sesquoxide. Germanium dioxide is not safe.

Recommended Dosage: 100 mcg per day.

IODINE

Although it will not correct thyroid conditions, *iodine* promotes good thyroid metabolism and helps in the production of thyroid hormones. There is about 30 mg of iodine naturally present in the body, and you should take in an additional 150 mcg per day—which is the RDA. Sea vegetables like kelp, nori, and hijiki are high in iodine, but these should be consumed only in moderation, as eating too many can result in an excess of iodine. Megadoses of any substance, even essential minerals, are unhealthy, as they throw your metabolism off balance. Iodine is found in most mineral formulas.

Recommended Dosage: 150 mcg per day.

IRON

Iron is the "heme" in hemoglobin, which is the component of the blood that gives it its red color. It is also required for the production of red blood cells. Red meat is rich in iron, which is also found in poultry, organ meats, fortified cereals, beans, nuts, seeds, and some vegetables in smaller amounts. Although the average American diet is very high in red meat, iron deficiency is common. High blood levels of iron are rare and usually caused by an inability to excrete unneeded iron effectively rather than excessive intake. Women are more prone to low iron levels than men, so RDAs differ; for females, it is 18 mg, and for males, 10 mg. Quality iron supplements contain the female RDA. Iron sulfate, fumarate, and gluconate are all good supplement choices.

Recommended Dosage: 18 mg per day.

MAGNESIUM

This mineral plays a role in energy production and regulates the body's levels of calcium, copper, potassium, vitamin D, and zinc. It is also needed by each of your organs to ensure their proper function. Most American diets are very deficient in magnesium, which is found in whole grains, leafy green vegetables, nuts, legumes, and some types of seeds, such as pumpkin and squash seeds. In fact, most Americans take in only half of the needed amount, which is about 600 mg per day—400 mg from dietary sources and the remaining 200 mg from supplements. Magnesium is beneficial for conditions like diabetes, asthma, high blood pressure, osteoporosis, and PMS. Magnesium citrate, lactate, and oxide are all effective forms.

Recommended Dosage: 600 mg per day (200 mg from supplements and 400 from dietary sources).

MANGANESE

A small amount (20 mg) of this trace mineral is naturally present in the body, found mostly in the bones, kidneys, pancreas, and liver. In addition to its role in metabolism, *manganese* aids in calcium absorption, blood sugar regulation, brain function, and the formation of connective tissues. It is also a basic component of the enzyme superoxide dismutase (SOD), which acts as an antioxidant. There has been a significant amount of research on the health benefits of manganese. It is plentiful in many foods, especially whole grains, beans, nuts, seeds, and leafy green vegetables. The RDA (2 mg) was established only recently. When supplementing with manganese, use either sulfates or oxides.

Recommended Dosage: 2 mg per day.

MOLYBDENUM

This element is present in the body and many foods, and is commonly used by farmers and gardeners in fertilizers and animal feed. Even though *molybdenum* is a heavy metal, it is completely safe and nontoxic. Deficiency is not a widespread problem, as humans do not require the mineral in large quantities. Good dietary sources include legumes, grains, leafy green vegetables, and nuts. The RDA for molybdenum, which is found in most mineral supplements, is 75 mcg.

Recommended Dosage: 75 mcg per day.

NICKEL

Small amounts of *nickel*, another overlooked trace mineral, are required by the body for functions such as energy production and protein circulation. Important to human and animal nutrition, nickel is found in foods such as nuts, soybeans, and oatmeal. Yet little research has been done on the benefits of nickel or the problems that may result from a nickel deficiency. Nickel is rarely found in mineral formulas, despite the fact that deficiency is common. You need only about 100 mcg per day. Regular salts, such as chlorides and sulfates, are effective.

Recommended Dosage: 100 mcg per day.

RUBIDIUM

Rubidium is not a trace element, but rather a basic mineral essential to human nutrition. And yet the importance of this element is almost always ignored. There is no official RDA for rubidium, and it is hardly ever found in mineral supplements, but research suggests that the mineral helps maintain hormone balance, glucose regulation, and iron absorption. It may also benefit people who suffer from depression. Good dietary sources include fruits, vegetables, poultry, and fish. The best supplement form to use is rubidium chloride. Rubidium deficiency has not been demonstrated.

Recommended Dosage: 500 mcg per day.

SELENIUM

Selenium is essential to good health but required only in small amounts—intake should not exceed 200 mcg per day. Although it has been mostly ignored—an official RDA of 70 mcg was set only recently—selenium has a number of important functions. It acts as an antioxidant and plays a role in thyroid health and immunity. Low levels of selenium are associated with a number of medical conditions, including heart disease, arthritis, diabetes, and some types of cancer. The best food sources of selenium are Brazil nuts, whole grains, brewer's yeast, wheat germ, fish, and shellfish. Refined foods, as well as soil, are deficient in selenium. Use a supplement that contains selenium in the form of chelates, which have better absorbability.

Recommended Dosage: 70 to 200 mcg per day.

SILICON

A vital but overlooked mineral, *silicon* makes up an amazing 33 percent of the earth's crust. It has been studied as a treatment for a number of conditions, including osteoporosis, Alzheimer's disease, heart disease, and digestive disorders. In addition, research has found that silicon aids in bone and joint metabolism, as well as calcium absorption. Unfortunately, most supplement manufacturers do not yet include this inexpensive essential element in their formulas, and there is no official RDA. Still, be sure to choose a supplement formula that contains silicon, which can be in the form of silicic acid (silica gel). Do not buy products containing horsetail, which is not a good source of silicon.

Recommended Dosage: 10 mg per day.

STRONTIUM

Strontium is another very important trace element with very good science behind it, even though there is no official RDA. This mineral is necessary for strong bones and joints, and it aids in calcium absorption. The average American diet is deficient in strontium, and you will almost never find it in mineral formulas. Therefore, it's important that you find a complete mineral supplement that contains it. The most common form found in dietary supplements is strontium chloride. Chelates and aspartates are also good choices. Look for a product that contains 1,000 mcg. Do not confuse strontium with strontium-90, which is its radioactive form.

Recommended Dosage: 1,000 mcg (1 mg) per day.

TIN

Tin is a trace mineral that is believed to play a role in many biological processes. Human studies have shown that low tin levels are common in people with various medical conditions and diseases. Unfortunately, the FDA limits the daily dose of tin to 30 mcg, and it is rarely found in mineral formulas. Tin is available in supplement form as tin chloride and tin sulfate, both of which are effective and well absorbed.

Recommended Dosage: 100 mcg per day.

VANADIUM

The importance of this trace mineral was ignored until very recently. There is still no official RDA for *vanadium*, even though scientists around the world have found that it is vital for human and animal health. Vanadium has specific, known health benefits for diabetics, as research has shown that it may help lower blood sugar and increase insulin sensitivity. It is found mainly in whole grains, so most people in the United States and other Western countries do not take in a sufficient amount through the diet. Vanadium is also rarely contained in mineral formulas. The best supplement forms are vanadium chelate and vanadium sulfate (vandal sulfate). Do not take vanadium in large amounts, as it is a heavy element and can cause toxicity in the body. An ideal dose is 1 mg (1,000 mcg) per day; it is irresponsible to take larger doses.

Recommended Dosage: 1 mg per day.

ZINC

Found in meats, whole grains, and beans, *zinc* is an essential mineral contained in nearly all mineral supplements. Approximately 2.5 g exists in the body, and half of this amount is stored in the muscles. The official RDA for women is 8 mg per day and for men, 11 mg per day, but deficiency is fairly common among alcoholics, elderly people, and the poor, who tend to eat foods lacking in nutrition. The published research on zinc is simply overwhelming. This mineral ensures the proper function of hundreds of enzymes—including superoxide dismutase (an antioxidant) and those involved in the carbohydrate and protein metabolism—and it plays a role in immunity, insulin regulation, and wound healing. Despite its benefits, dosage amounts should never exceed 50 mg per day, since consuming large amounts can result in toxicity. Take supplements that contain zinc citrate, zinc oxide, or zinc sulfate.

Recommended Dosage: 10 mg per day.

OTHER MINERALS

Since trace elements are present in such tiny amounts in the body and various foods, it is difficult to study them and determine the specific roles they play in your health. *Barium,* for example, is essential, but human deficiencies have not been reported. *Lithium* is also an essential mineral, and megadoses are used to treat mania and depressive disorders. Most people probably have a sufficient amount of lithium in their diet. Other elements that need further study or are currently being researched include:

- Cerium
- Dysprosium
- Erbium
- Europium
- Gadolinium
- Indium
- Lanthanum
- Neodymium
- Praseodymium
- Samarium
- Thulium
- Titanium
- Tungsten
- Yttrium

Keep in mind that not every mineral has medicinal value or health benefits. Gold, silver, platinum, and palladium, for example, do not play any role in health. Moreover, there are minerals that are actually harmful, including lead, cadmium, aluminum, arsenic, mercury, and thallium. Lead is the most toxic heavy metal for humans, followed by aluminum. Arsenic, cadmium, mercury and thallium account for less human toxicity. Eating well, restricting your calorie intake, exercising, and fasting every week are good ways to lower the levels of these toxic metals in your body. Taking 3 g of sodium alginate (see page 127), a seaweed extract, per day for six to twelve months is an effective way to completely rid your body of these metals.

CHOOSING MINERAL SUPPLEMENTS

Hardly any mineral supplements contain all the essential elements listed in this chapter. The key to buying a quality product is to read labels. If it's not on the label, it's not in the bottle. Be sure to note every single mineral in the product, along with the specified amounts. If the provided dose is significantly lower than the RDA, you can rest assured that the supplement is a waste of money. In addition, never buy "proprietary formulas," which are supplements packed with "filler" minerals. Manufacturers of proprietary formulas are not legally obligated to disclose every substance they put in their products. Overall, you should only buy a supplement if it contains most of the essential minerals in meaningful amounts. A simple Internet search can lead you to a complete quality product.

CONCLUSION

Scientists do not yet have all the answers when it comes to minerals and nutrition. Undoubtedly, more essential minerals will be found in the future and, hopefully, a more affordable and realistic method of testing mineral levels will soon be developed. In the mean time, be sure to take each mineral discussed in this chapter, along with the supplements in Chapter 16 (see page 117). Remember that minerals work synergistically, which means you must meet your recommended requirement for each element. By choosing the right mineral supplements and following a healthy diet of whole natural foods, you will be well on your way to reversing your mineral deficiency.

ESSENTIAL MINERALS		
Mineral	**Optimal Daily Intake**	**Considerations**
Boron	3 mg	Take as boric acid or boric citrate.
Calcium	500 mg (250 mg from supplements and 250 mg from dietary sources)	Whole grains, green leafy vegetables, beans, sprouts, and soy foods are better dietary sources of calcium than dairy products. As a supplement, calcium should be taken as calcium citrate or calcium carbonate.
Cesium	100 mcg	Vital but overlooked element. Take 100 mcg daily.
Chromium	120 to 400 mcg	Use chelates, which are absorbed well by the body. Your daily dose should not exceed 400 mg.
Cobalt	25 mcg	Take in the form of methylcobalamin.
Copper	2 mg	Copper citrate, oxide, and gluconate are effective bioavailable forms. Do not exceed the recommended dose.
Gallium	100 mcg	Gallium nitrate is the best form to take.
Germanium	100 mcg	Germanium dioxide is not safe. Use chelates or germanium sesquoxide.
Iodine	150 mcg	Found in many sea vegetables, iodine supports thyroid function and is contained in most mineral formulas.
Iron	18 mg	Quality iron supplements contain the recommended dose for women (18 mg), not the recommendation for men, which is slightly lower (10 mg). Iron sulfate, fumarate, and gluconate are acceptable supplement forms.
Magnesium	600 mg (400 mg from dietary sources and 200 mg from supplements)	Abundant in whole grains, leafy greens, legumes, nuts, and some seeds. The best supplement forms are magnesium citrate, lactate, and oxide.
Manganese	2 mg	Use sulfates or oxides. Manganese is also naturally present in whole grains, beans, nuts, and seeds.

Mineral	Optimal Daily Intake	Considerations
Molybdenum	75 mcg	Found in most mineral formulas as well as legumes, grains, nuts, and leafy green vegetables.
Nickel	100 mcg	Most people take in a sufficient amount through foods like nuts, soybeans, and oatmeal. The best supplement forms are chlorides and sulfates.
Rubidinum	500 mcg	Research suggests this mineral helps maintain hormone and blood sugar balance, and improves iron absorption. Take rubidinum chloride.
Selenium	70 to 200 mcg	Use a supplement that contains selenium in the form of chelates, which have better absorbability.
Silicon	10 mg	Take silicic acid. Do not buy products that contain horsetail.
Strontium	1,000 mcg	Strontium chloride is the form most commonly found in supplements, but chelates and aspartates are also acceptable.
Tin	100 mcg	Low levels are common in people with a broad range of medical conditions, yet tin is rarely found in mineral formulas. Tin chloride and tin sulfate are effective and well absorbed.
Vanadium	1 mg	An important trace element vital to blood sugar metabolism.
Zinc	10 mg	Helps with immunity, insulin regulation, and wound healing. Never exceed 50 mg per day.

Seven Steps
to Natural Health

The following steps are of vital importance for a long and healthy life. With these seven steps, you can prevent and treat "incurable" diseases like cancer, diabetes, heart disease, osteoporosis, arthritis, and others naturally without drugs or invasive medical procedures like surgery and chemotherapy. You can also shed excess weight, fight obesity, and alleviate undesirable symptoms of menopause and premenstrual syndrome, all of which are affecting increasing numbers of women in the Western world. Every medical condition discussed in this book can be prevented, treated, or reversed with these seven essential steps. Along with stress reduction techniques like prayer and meditation, incorporate the guidelines below into your everyday life.

1. Follow an American macrobiotic whole grain-based diet. Diet is the single most crucial factor in achieving and maintaining good health. Diet prevents and cures disease. Everything else is secondary.

2. Take the proven nutritional supplements highlighted in Chapters 16 and 17 (see pages 117 and 131) to enhance the positive effects of your diet. Remember, if you are at least forty years of age, you should take all of the listed vitamins, minerals, and other nutrients.

3. Balance your hormone levels. If you are deficient in a certain hormone, take bioidentical hormone supplements. Excessive levels of a hormone can be lowered with diet and lifestyle. You can also easily and inexpensively measure your basic hormones using at-home saliva tests or an online lab.

4. Exercise regularly, even if you walk for just thirty minutes every day. Exercise is essential to your physical, mental, and emotional well-being. An ideal workout routine consists of both aerobic and resistance training.

5. Fast one day per week, drinking only water from dinner to dinner. Fasting is one of the most powerful healing methods known. You can also join Young Again's two-day fast, which takes place on the last weekend of every month. More information is available at www.youngagain.org.

6. Avoid prescription drugs. Exceptions are temporary antibiotics, pain medication in the event of an emergency, and necessary medications, such as insulin for type 1 diabetics.

7. End bad habits like drinking alcohol and using recreational drugs. You should also limit desserts and coffee consumption. You don't have to be a saint, but you do need to be responsible when it comes to matters of your health.

Conclusion

As you may have noted, the information contained in this book is vastly different from the information commonly circulated by doctors and mainstream medical resources. For years, it seems, the study of women's health has played second fiddle to the study of men's health. For decades, whatever results came out of male-oriented research was quickly applied to women without a second thought. Not only that, but in the male-dominated profession of medicine, male doctors were always presumed to know best—whether it was about reproduction, menstrual cycles, or menopause—while women were told what to do and expected to follow orders. Too many times were women told things like, "It's all in your head" or "These tranquilizers should help." Even worse, female patients were often provided with out-of-date information for many serious conditions.

Today, things are changing. New studies are now focusing solely on women and providing crucial information that could save a woman's life, such as how to recognize a heart attack, which can be very different from a male heart attack. Women are now not afraid to question their doctors or learn about safe alternatives when it comes to their health. That is the reason behind this book. Instead of being told what to do without question, you need to know the facts and take responsibility for your own health. The more you know, the better prepared you will be to regain your health through a more natural method that is in tune with your body.

Reading this book, however, is only the first step. The information provided here will not work unless you take action. The door may now be open, but you need to take the next steps and learn as much as you can. Once you do, handing over your well-being to someone else will no longer be an option.

Wishing you the best of health and a long life.

Recommended Reading

FASTING

Bragg, Patricia and Paul C. Bragg. *The Miracle of Fasting.* 50th ed. Bragg Health Sciences, 2004.

Bueno-Aguer, Lee. *Fast Your Way to Health.* New Kensington, PA: Whitaker House, 1991.

Cott, Allan. *Fasting: The Ultimate Diet.* New York: Hastings House, 2006.

Fuhrman, Joel and Neal D. Barnard. *Fasting and Eating for Health.* New York: St. Martin's Press, 1995.

FEMALE CANCER, HYSTERECTOMY, AND MENOPAUSE

Cutler, Winnifred. *Hysterectomy: Before & After.* New York: Harper & Row, 1988.

Hufnagel, Vicki and Susan K. Golant. *No More Hysterectomies;* revised edition. New York: Plume, 1995.

Kradjigan, Robert. *Save Yourself from Breast Cancer.* New York: Berkley Books, 1994.

Lee, John, Jesse Hanley, and Virginia Hopkins. *What Your Doctor May Not Tell You About Premenopause.* New York: Warner Books, 1999.

Lee, John, and Virginia Hopkins. *What Your Doctor May Not Tell You About Menopause.* New York: Warner Books, 2004.

Payer, Lynn. *How to Avoid a Hysterectomy.* New York: Pantheon Books, 1988.

Stokes, Naomi Miller. *The Castrated Woman: What Your Doctor Won't Tell You About Hysterectomy.* London: Franklin Watts, 1986.

Strausz, Ivan. *You Don't Need a Hysterectomy.* New York: De Capo Press, 2001.

Stanley West, *The Hysterectomy Hoax*. Chester, NJ: New Decade, Inc., 2002.

GENERAL HEALTH AND WELLNESS

Barnard, Neal. *Eat Right, Live Longer: Using the Natural Power of Foods to Age-Proof Your Body*. New York: Three Rivers Press, 2001.

——. *Food For Life: How the New Four Food Groups Can Save Your Life*. New York: Three Rivers Press, 1993.

——. *Live Longer, Live Better*. Book Publishing Company, 1999. (Audio.)

——. *Turn Off the Fat Genes: The Revolutionary Guide to Losing Weight*. New York: Three Rivers Press, 2001.

Null, Gary. *Get Healthy Now! A Complete Guide to Prevention, Treatment, and Healthy Living*. New York: Seven Stories Press, 2001.

——. *The Seven Steps to Perfect Health*. New York: ibooks, Inc., 2001.

——. *The Vegetarian Handbook: Eating Right for Total Health*. New York: St. Martin's Press, 1996.

Ornish, Dean. *Eat More, Weigh Less: Dr. Dean Ornish's Life Choice Program for Losing Weight Safely While Eating Abundantly*. New York: Quill, 2001.

——. *Program for Reversing Heart Disease*. New York: Ballantine Books, 1996.

Powter, Susan. *Food*. New York: Pocket Books, 1995.

——. *Stop the Insanity*. New York: Pocket Books, 1993.

Shintani, Terry. *The Good Carbohydrate Revolution: A Proven Program for Low-Maintenance Weight Loss and Optimum Health*. New York: Pocket Books, 2002.

——. *The Hawaii Diet*. New York: Pocket Books, 1999.

Walford, Roy. *The 120 Year Diet: How to Double Your Vital Years*. New York: Simon & Schuster, 1986. Reprint, 2000.

——. *Maximum Life Span*. New York: W.W. Norton & Company, 2006.

About the Author

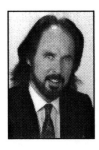 Roger Mason is an internationally known research chemist who studies natural health and longevity. He has written ten different unique and cutting-edge books about his findings. He sold Beta Prostate® in 2011, walked away from radio and TV, and formed a charitable trust. He lives with his wife and dog in Wilmington, NC, where they run Young Again Products. You can read his weekly newsletter, books, and more than 300 articles for free at www.YoungAgain.org.

Index

OTHER TITLES BY ROGER MASON

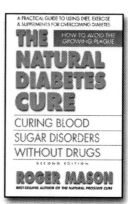

$9.95 • 978-0-7570-0369-1

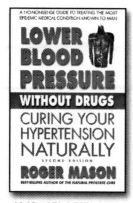

$9.95 • 978-0-7570-0366-0

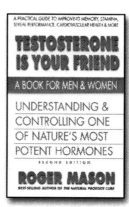

$9.95 • 978-0-7570-0371-4

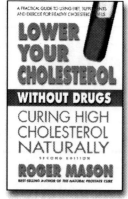

$9.95 • 978-0-7570-0367-7

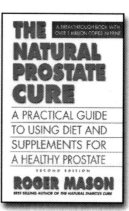

$9.95 • 978-0-7570-0370-7